IUD Technology

Progress in Contraceptive Delivery Systems

Volume I	Biodegradables and Delivery Systems for Contraception
Volume II	IUDs and Family Planning
Volume III	IUD Pathology and Management
Volume IV	IUD Technology

see p. 197 for details

Progress in Contraceptive Delivery Systems

Series Editor: E. S. E. Hafez

VOLUME IV

IUD TECHNOLOGY

EDITORS

E. S. E. Hafez
Detroit, Michigan
USA

A. J. M. Audebert
Bordeaux
France

MTP PRESS LIMITED
LANCASTER · BOSTON · THE HAGUE
International Medical Publishers

This volume is dedicated to Margaret Sanger (1879–1966). Margaret Sanger was the founder and first President of the International Planned Parenthood Federation. Her autobiography is published by Dover Publications, Inc. (Photograph courtesy of Planned Parenthood – World Population, 810 Seventh Avenue, New York, NY 10019, USA)

Published in the UK and Europe by
MTP Press Limited
Falcon House
Lancaster, England

British Library Cataloguing in Publication Data

IUD technology.—(Progress in contraceptive
delivery systems; v. 4)
1. Intrauterine contraceptives
I. Hafez, E. S. E.
II. Audebert, A. III. Series
613.91'435 RG137.3

ISBN 0-85200-356-0

Published in the USA by
MTP Press
A division of Kluwer Boston Inc
190 Old Derby Street
Hingham, MA 02043, USA

Library of Congress Cataloging in Publication Data

Main entry under title:

IUD technology.

(Progress in contraceptive delivery systems; v. 4)
"Papers at the International Symposium on IUD Technology which was held from July 3–5, 1980, in Bordeaux, France"—Foreword.
Includes bibliographical references and index.
1. Intrauterine contraceptives—Congresses.
I. Hafez, E. S. E., 1922–II. II. Audebert, A. III. International Symposium on IUD Technology (1980: Bordeaux, France) IV. Title: I.U.D. technology. V. Series.
RG137.3.I9 613.9'435 81-20757

ISBN 0-85200-356-0 AACR2

Phototypesetting by Georgia Origination, Liverpool
Printed in Great Britain by Butler & Tanner Ltd, Frome and London

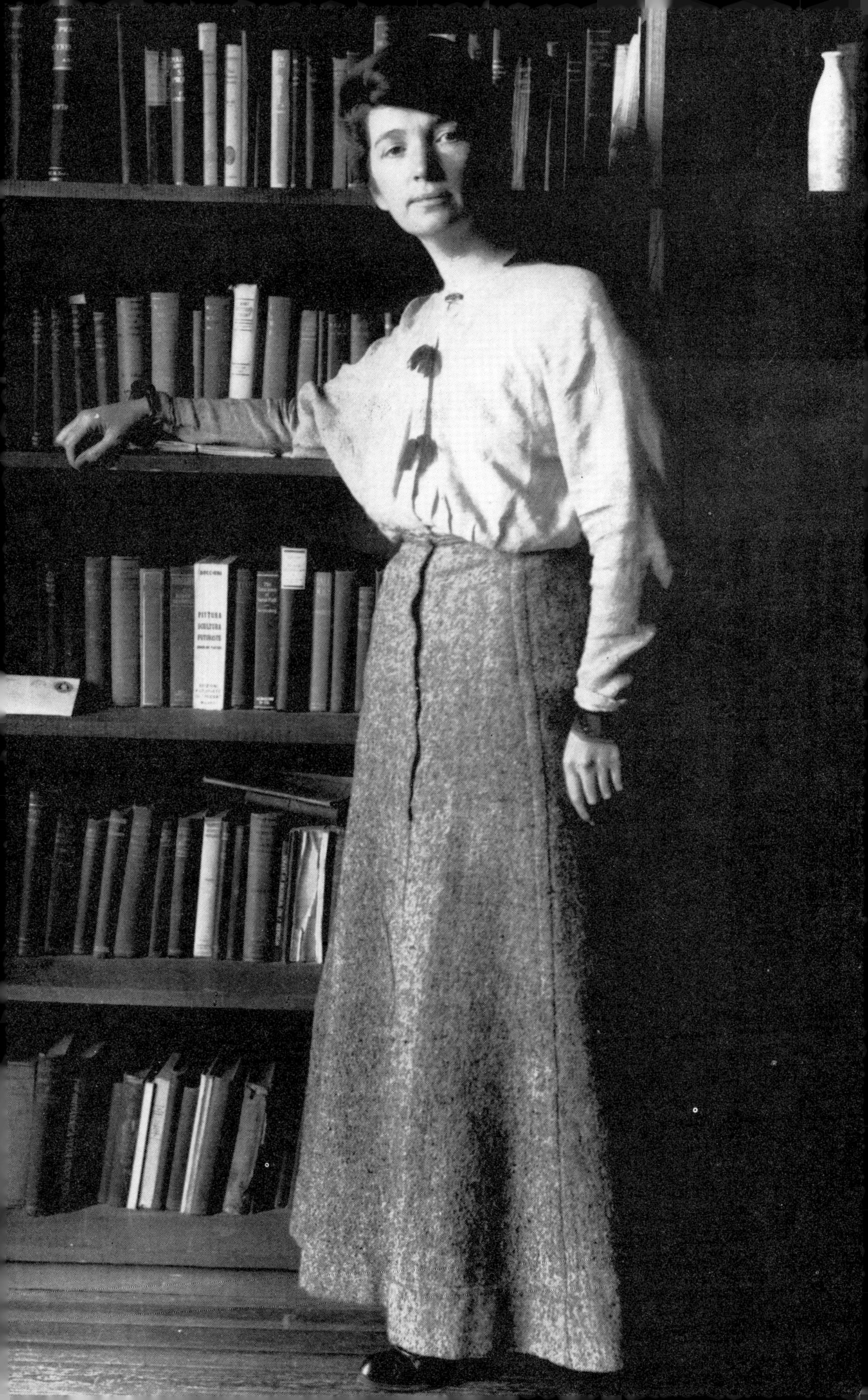

Contents

List of contributors

A. H. ANSARI
Department of Obstetrics and Gynecology
Georgia Baptist Medical Center
Atlanta Fertility Institute, P.C.
340 Boulevard, N.E.
Atlanta, Georgia 30312, USA

V. M. ANSARI
Atlanta Fertility Institute, P.C.
340 Boulevard, N.E.
Atlanta, Georgia 30312, USA

G. S. BERGER
Departments of Obstetrics and Gynecology and Maternal and Child Health
University of North Carolina
Schools of Medicine and Public Health
Chapel Hill Fertility Services
109 Conner Drive
Chapel Hill, NC 27514, USA

B. BOURGEOIS
Centre Carreire
121 Rue de la Bechade, 121
33076 Bordeaux, France

Y. GIBOR
Gynecology and Infertility Clinic
25 Brei Noshe Street
Tel Aviv, Israel

J. C. GOODPASTURE
Department of Obstetrics and Gynecology
University Hospitals
Hufelandstrasse 55
4300 Essen 1, West Germany

E. S. E. HAFEZ
Department of Gynecology and Obstetrics
The C. S. Mott Center for Human Growth and Development
Wayne State University School of Medicine
Detroit, Michigan 48201, USA

A. A. HASPELS
Department of Obstetrics and Gynecology
University Hospital
Catharijnesingel 101
3511 GV Utrecht
The Netherlands

H. M. HASSON
Department of Obstetrics and Gynecology
Grant Hospital of Chicago, and Northwestern University Medical School, 2424 N. Clark St
Chicago, Illinois 60614, USA

LIST OF CONTRIBUTORS

M. F. HAYES
Department of Gynecology and Obstetrics
Wayne State University School of Medicine
The C. S. Mott Center for Human Growth and Development
275 E. Hancock, Detroit, Michigan 48201, USA

L. G. KEITH
Department of Obstetrics and Gynecology
Northwestern University Medical School and the Prentice Women's Hospital and Maternity Center
Chicago, Illinois, USA

M. LEVRIER
College de Gynecologie de Bordeaux et du Sud-Ouest
Genevieve Roux
24 avenue de Lattre de Tassigny
33400 Talence, France

H. LUDWIG
Department of Obstetrics and Gynecology
University Hospitals
Hufelandstrasse 55
4300 Essen 1, West Germany

K. S. MOGHISSI
Department of Gynecology and Obstetrics
Wayne State University School of Medicine,
The C. S. Mott Center for Human Growth and Development
275 E. Hancock, Detroit
Michigan 48201, USA

M. NOHLEN
Department of Obstetrics and Gynecology
University Hospitals
Hufelandstrasse 55
4300 Essen 1, West Germany

W. A. A. van OS,
St Elisabeth's de Groote Gasthuis
P.O. Box 417
2000 AK Haarlem, The Netherlands

M. ROBINSON
ALZA Corporation
950 Page Mill Road
Palo Alto, California 94304, USA

J. J. SCIARRA
Department of Obstetrics and Gynecology
Northwestern University Medical School
Chicago, Illinois 60611, USA

A. SCOMMEGNA
Department of Obstetrics and Gynecology
Michael Reese Hospital and Medical Center
29th Street and Ellis Avenue
Chicago, Illinois 60616, USA

S. SHARRETT
Grant Hospital of Chicago
550 W. Webster Avenue
Chicago, Illinois 60614, USA

P. F. TAUBER
Department of Obstetrics and Gynecology
University Hospitals
Hufelandstrasse 55
4300 Essen 1, West Germany

M. R. VAN SANTEN
Department of Obstetrics and Gynecology
University Hospital
P.O. Box 16250
3500 CG Utrecht
The Netherlands

B. VEIL
Providencia 2457,
Apart. 415
Santiago
Chile

R. WEINSTEIN
International Planned Parenthood Federation
Western Hemisphere Region
New York City, New York, USA

LIST OF CONTRIBUTORS

G. I. ZATUCHNI
Department of Obstetrics and Gynecology
Northwestern University Medical School, Room 1040
303 East Superior Street
Chicago, Illinois 60611, USA

J. ZIPPER
Departmento de Fisiologia y Biofisica
Universidad de Chile
Escuela de Medicina
Casilla 6524, Santiago, Chile

Foreword

Science and research continues to strive for the totality of means used to provide appropriate methods necessary for human contraceptive sustenance and comfort. Searching for total safety and effectiveness of contraceptives continually stimulates new research. Most methods presently under study are used or could be used if made available, or are at a stage of development where their usefulness is likely to be assessed over the next few years.

In particular, this volume deals with the widespread application of intrauterine contraceptive devices - the IUD - which did not occur actively until the 1960s. Since then, the devices in existence have made remarkable improvements. The contributors to this volume presented their papers at the International Symposium on *IUD Technology* which was held from July 3-5, 1980, in Bordeaux, France. All research efforts have strived to make IUDs as effective as possible while at the same time minimizing the existence of side-effects. One approach to improving the effectiveness, safety and acceptability is to develop methods of delivery that provide programmed medication. This is based on knowing that side-effects are generally dose dependent and that the degree of risk changes in proportion to the dose. The preferred dose is one that evokes contraception with minimal risk.

To promote widespread successful application, the physician must put the benefit-risk ratio of the IUD in a proper perspective. By obtaining a thorough knowledge of the practical results with all available devices and by utilizing the objective scientific data accumulated in the process of development, the physician can then adequately provide appropriate contraception to all those desiring it.

This volume concentrates on present knowledge obtained in the areas of inert and medicated IUDs, applications and complications of IUDs, and IUDs and family planning. To develop long-acting contraceptive systems, the application of more sophisticated technology is required, as is a wider diversity of technological expertise. The multidisciplinary approach to research requires centralization of advanced expertise and a broad funding base to be totally effective.

The editors would like to express their sincere appreciation to all the contributors of this volume, who so meticulously prepared their chapters and who share in the general goal of providing safe and effective contraception to the world. Thanks are also due to Jackie Mucci, who assisted in the editing and assembling of this volume; to Jackie Smieska for her helpful assistance; and to MTP Press for their fine preparation of this publication.

January 1982
Detroit, Michigan, USA

E. S. E. HAFEZ
Series Editor

Part I
INERT AND MEDICATED IUDs

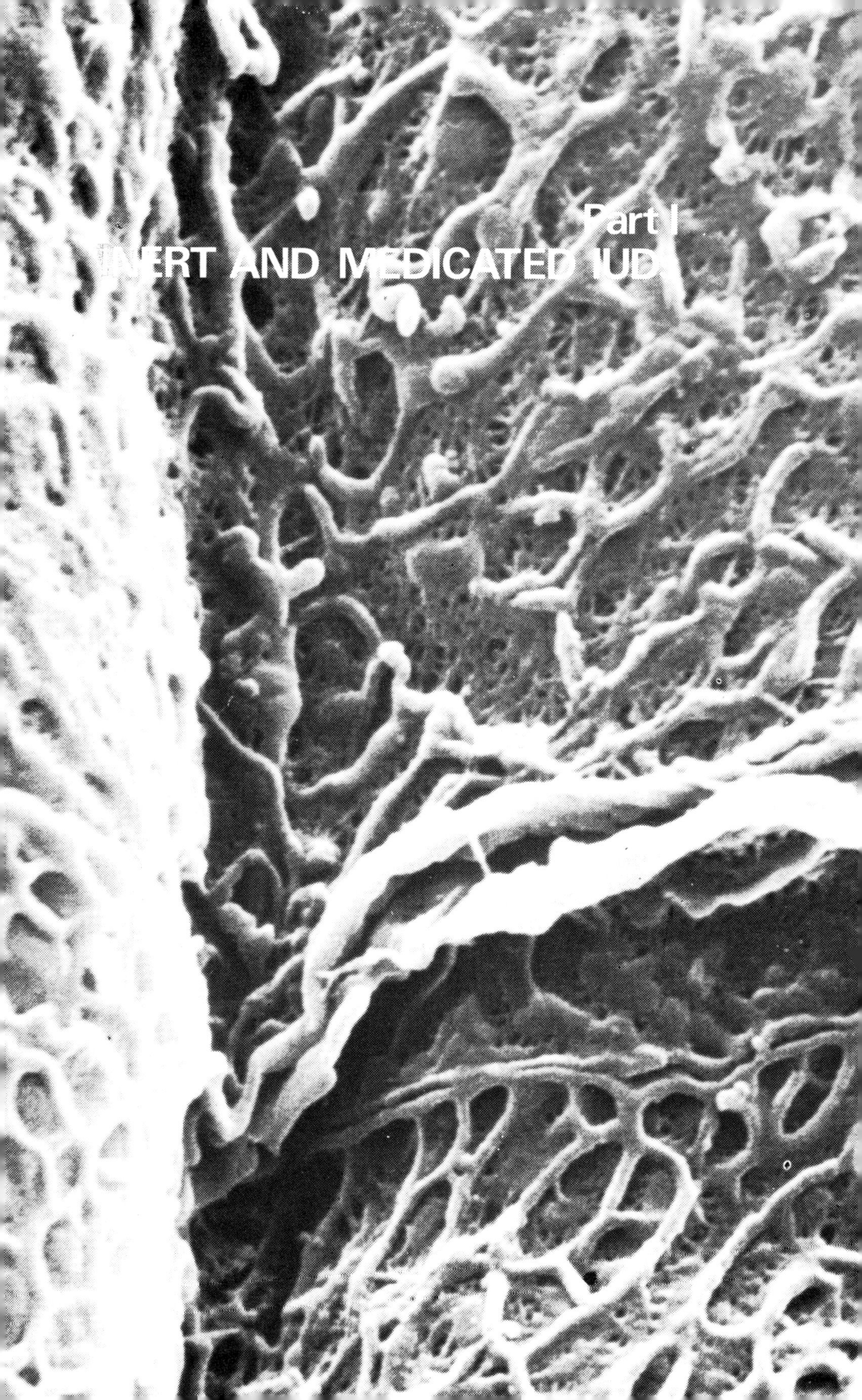

1
Fertility regulation and modern technology

E. S. E. HAFEZ

Fertility regulation and family planning are both essential factors in developing a 'natural economy', maintaining the 'quality of life', and protecting both maternal and child health. Family planning is encouraged in densely populated areas, whereas appropriate measures are adopted to increase the population in sparsely populated minority areas. People will be encouraged to marry late, and families will be encouraged to plan only one or two children at most, with a 3-year gap between children (Figure 1.1).

A dramatic culture revolution now exists which includes an overall increase in cohabitation and a decrease in birth rate as well as a natural increase in growth rate, and decrease in death rate. An equilibrium between these factors is highly critical in maintaining a natural economy and quality of life. In both men and women, sexual behavior in middle age is greatly influenced by socio-cultural background. Cohabitation is common in various parts of the world and is becoming more popular. Concepts and methods of contraception therefore vary accordingly.

In parts of Africa, as elsewhere, a woman is not expected to have any more children after she has a married daughter, or otherwise becomes a grandmother. In parts of Hindu India, the idea of manhood may be to marry at age 25, to have 25 years of fertile life and then to abstain from sex thereafter. As men often marry younger brides, it is not uncommon for women to abstain from intercourse well before they reach the end of their fertile years. In some parts of Asia, coital frequency in couples between ages 40 and 50 is significantly lower than among those in the West.

The impact of contraception on population growth varies considerably in different countries as a result of various factors such as culture, religion, socio-economic condition, education, general health and standard of living. These differences are apparent when contrasting the Middle East with Latin America; and Africa with China. One of the most important demographic events in human history is that China has cut its birth and growth rates approximately in half during the last decade. Family planning in China has

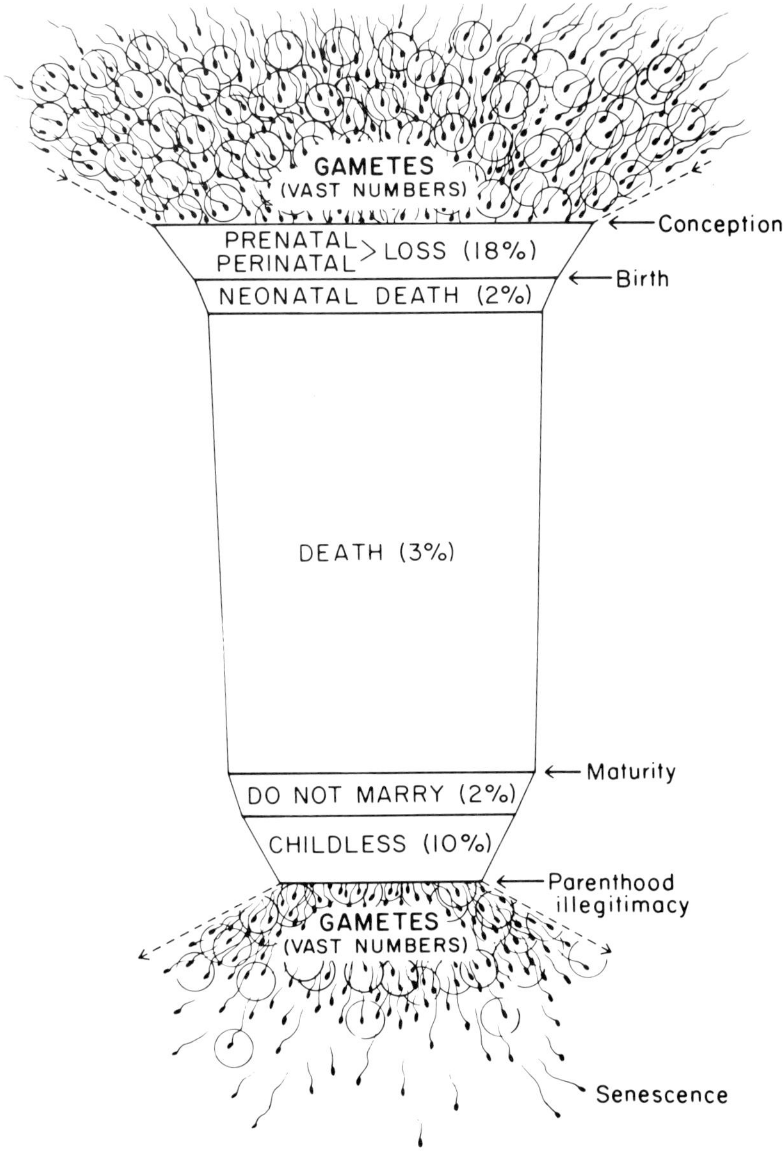

Figure 1.1 Diagram of life cycle, showing effect of sexual reproduction on variability. Gametes are produced in large numbers and suffer a large random loss. Prenatal and perinatal loss is estimated as 18%, neonatal death as 5%, and death before sexual maturity as 3%. Of survivors, 2% do not marry before the end of childbearing age. Of those who do marry, 10% are childless (From Sladen, B. K. and Bang, F. B. (eds.) (1969). *Biology of Populations: The Bioligical Basis of Public Health*, p. 188. (New York: American Elsevier).

been successful due to: (1) delay of marriage and reproduction until at least the mid-twenties; (2) full availability of all the most effective contraceptive methods - IUDs, oral contraceptives, condoms, voluntary sterilization, and abortion; and (3) intense education and peer pressure for planned and reduced reproduction.

CONTRACEPTIVE REVOLUTION

Since the perfect contraceptive has not yet been developed, research continues. Attempts for improving contraceptive methods include new synthentic antifertility drugs for both male and female as well as the ability for women to easily and accurately determine their own fertile period. During the last decade, over 1500 chemical entities have been developed and/or tested. Although new formulas are always being discovered, most are not pursued beyond animal testing. Some of these compounds may have high antifertility activity, but it is difficult to prove their effectiveness and safety. The method of administering contraceptives is also important in improving fertility regulation. By reducing the drug burden on the body, a greater degree of safety can be achieved by substituting naturally occurring steroids for synthetic ones. Consequently, considerable progress has been made in the area of contraceptive delivery systems.

Experimental attempts to develop devices that will occlude the vas deferens or fallopian tubes to permit temporary or easily reversed sterilization have been less successful.

WHO NEEDS CONTRACEPTION?

Contraception is most important for professional women, disturbed women, teenagers, women in developing countries and for women who reach their desired number of children. A career women in her 30s who is professionally successful and financially secure may request contraception to maintain her present independence without having the fear of pregnancy. In developing countries, a woman's career may hold higher priorities for the betterment of the country, rather than choosing a family.

Disturbed women

The disturbed woman whether by the trauma of rape, fear of abortion, or perhaps mentally ill, may not desire the birth of a child and would therefore require some contraceptive method to minimize this emotional stress. Realizing the impossibility of being able to adequately raise a child would also determine one's acceptance to contraceptives.

Teenagers

In today's society, most teenagers find themselves pregnant without being prepared for the psychological, physical, or financial outcome. Many of these teenagers are not informed of available contraceptive choices that exist, and are often unable to obtain them without parental consent. Consequently, pregnant teenagers may either resort to inadequate abortion clinics, excessive drugs or else give birth to the child and place it for adoption, or raise the child under strenuous conditions. Therefore, major emphasis should be placed on contraception, with accurate informants in the school system to provide the necessary knowledge to teenagers on various methods of choice.

Teenage pregnancy clinics do exist where a pregnant teenager (12–19 years old) can receive individual medical care and take part in group counseling sessions while continuing their education in a supportive atmosphere throughout their pregnancy. Once the baby is born, the mother and baby can return to the clinic for monthly visits with the social worker or psychologist. Support and guidance are offered by the social worker for continuing the mother's education if interrupted by the pregnancy.

Contraceptive counseling is most essential in school systems to advise and inform both teenage males and females of various contraceptive methods available, their effectiveness and side-effects. During the last decade, there has been an extraordinary increase in teenage promiscuity and sexual activity. In the USA, nearly half of all out-of-wedlock births are attributed to teenagers, and up to two-thirds of these are unwanted and unplanned births. Due to the rapidly changing sexual mores, the teenager feels trapped and confused by peer pressure, uncertainty, timidity, ignorance and misinformation. Consequently, the younger patient needs and deserves thorough counseling underlined with compassion, reassurance, and trust in many areas. These areas may range from the basic facts of reproduction and fertility to more serious subjects like venereal disease and consequences of pregnancy. Contraception is definitely a sensitive and controversial issue.

Due to the unavailability of proportionally sized IUDs for nulliparous teenagers, IUD use is restricted to such special cases as: (1) girls of unfavorable socio-economic background and/or uncontrollable ways of life; (2) mentally retarded girls without efficient supervision; (3) emotionally unstable girls with infrequent, irregular intercourse; and (4) where hormonal contraceptives are contraindicated. The small uterus of adolescents does not always support a normal-sized IUD.

MENSTRUATION AND CONTRACEPTION

A regular menstrual cycle reassures women whether they are pregnant or not. Consequently, any acceptable method of contraception must maintain a regular menstrual pattern. If regular menstruation is not important, a whole range of new methods of contraception will reduce the number of periods a woman has each year. This could prove to be an attraction rather than a deterrent to its use.

CONTRACEPTION FOR MIDDLE-AGED WOMEN

Owing to various social trends, fertility changes with age. In Europe, the birth rate of women over 35 years of age is 50%. This figure differs from 30% some 150 years ago. There are couples over the age of 35 who practice fertility control by sexual abstinence, contraception, or abortion.

The decrease in fertility at perimenopause may be due to the effects of age-related increases in the frequency of anovulatory cycles and inadequate luteal phases, and reduced frequency of intercourse. The incidence of certain genetic disorders and congenital malformations, especially chromosomal imbalance in the fetus, increases with age of the mother. There may also be an increase in the number of gene mutations and some environmental factors, especially the early maternal environment which may become deficient.

Two hundred years ago when there was no contraception, 30% of all births occurred in women over 35 years of age. Even a decade ago, one in 10 births occurred in women of this age group. Today it is less than one in 20. Contraception invariably begins with the control of pregnancy in older age groups. Contraception in middle-aged women is highly recommended because of the high rates of mortality and morbidity associated with pregnancy. This is an important reason for providing adequate advice on contraception where sexual relations do persist in older women. Oral contraceptives are not totally recommended and IUDs are more suitable and becoming more acceptable except when irregular bleeding is feared. Sterilization has become increasingly popular in avoiding the risks of morbidity and mortality associated with pregnancy in older women. Coitus interruptus is widely practiced, but has a high failure rate and some illnesses in women may be traced to its use. Use of the diaphragm accompanied with various contraceptive foams and jels is also widely accepted and effective if properly used. The rhythm method is highly ineffective due to irregular menstrual cycles which prevent exact timing of the safe period.

The age of menopause varies between populations but the average age of menopause ranges from 50 to 52 years. In developing countries, the age of menopause, although quite variable, is less than 44 years due to nutritional factors. The length of the menstrual cycle decreases with age. A transitional phase just before menopause begins, which varies in different women, is characterized by having both unusually long and short menstrual cycles. Contraception should continue through this phase if desired, until the onset of permanent menopausal absence of menstruation.

CONTRACEPTION FOR BREAST-FEEDING MOTHERS

During the puerperium, non-nursing women can feel free to choose hormonal oral contraceptives. This kind of contraception, however, is not advisable for women when breast feeding since it may interfere with milk production. The hormone itself or its metabolites may be ingested by the baby through the milk which could consequently produce growth disturbances. When breast feeding, IUDs can be used with confidence since it does not interfere with milk production or any hormonal changes. In the future, it may be possible to use special biodegradable IUDs which would distribute various nutrients to the suckling baby.

Breast feeding has a temporary contraceptive effect. It is not an efficient method of contraception because the resumption of ovulation and menstruation in lactating women shows a high individual variability. A contraceptive method may therefore be necessary during lactation, and oral contraceptives are widely used for this purpose. The transfer of exogenous contraceptive steroids into human milk during established lactation is being investigated.

Oral contraceptives taken by young women may result in adverse effects on the infant such as biological immaturity at birth. This danger of taking the pill too soon in life may especially endanger pre-term infants. However, since the start of oral contraception in the mid-fifties, there have been very few side-effects in breast-fed infants. There are indirect effects on the growth of babies due to decreased milk volume, but the only side-effect on infants is the development of gynecomastia in a very few cases.

ORAL CONTRACEPTIVES vs IUDs

Presently, oral contraceptives are the most popular reversible contraceptive method in the world. Predisposing factors related to high-risk rates of using OCs are hypertension, high cholesterol concentrations, circulatory diseases (arterial or venous disorders), diabetes, and obesity. Smoking cigarettes while taking the pill increases the risks further. Women tend to discontinue use of OCs when only a small supply is issued at the initial visit, and having to continuously visit their doctor for additional prescriptions. Use is also discontinued due to the daily aggravation of taking the pill at the same time, every day.

Knowledge of the IUD to the lay person is often inaccurate and misjudged. Various program personnel do not inform clients about the method's high degree of effectiveness. It is easier for family planning clinics to prescribe OCs rather than concern themselves with regular check-ups for IUDs. In some developing countries where contraceptives are negligible, i.e. Bangladesh, 200 per 100 000 women in each 5-year age group can be expected to die in childbirth. IUD users have substantially higher continuation rates than of any other contraceptive method used.

DISCOVERIES IN REPRODUCTIVE PHYSIOLOGY APPLICABLE TO FUTURE CONTRACEPTION

Extensive basic and clinical investigations have been conducted on various types of contraceptives (reviewed by Potts and Wood, 1972; Hafez, 1980; Hafez and van Os, 1980 a,b,c; Cunningham, *et al.* 1980). Several discoveries have been made in laboratories of basic sciences, such as folliculostatin – found to suppress FSH secretion by the pituitary in the female – oocyte maturation inhibitor, which acts to prevent the first meiotic division of the oocyte; and inhibin – a testicular hormone which inhibits secretion of FSH by pituitary cells without inhibiting LH secretion. Discovery of inhibin has added a new understanding of gonadal–pituitary feedback regulation. These major breakthroughs will be translated in the future into clinical application.

The following new approaches to fertility regulation should be used in the year 2000, based on recent advances in reproductive physiology:

(1) Structure and function of gonadotropins and their releasing hormones, their agonists, and antagonists.
(2) Reproductive hormone biosynthesis, metabolism, and mechanisms of action.

(3) Ovarian and testicular structure and function.
(4) Gamete maturation, transport, and fertilization.
(5) Discovery of an antibody to estrogen receptor.
(6) Presence of androgen-binding protein in testis.
(7) Presence of antigonadotropin of pineal gland.

BIODEGRADABLES

Since the 1950s, when Gregory Pincus developed contraceptive steroids, the oral administration of the pill has been the most common pharmacological approach to contraception. More recent developments have used injectable or implantable techniques based on sustained delivery systems. These first sustained drug delivery systems were generally prepared with bio-insert carriers (usually organic polymers). Although these systems generally work well, it is usually necessary or desirable to remove the inert carrier from the body after exhaustion of the drug reservoir. In recent years, therefore, there has been an increased interest in developing polymeric delivery systems that will biodegrade and disappear from the body site. Because of the ability to control the number and size of microcapsules injected, patients can be offered a 1-month course to determine whether the method is suitable before embarking on a 6-month or 1-year course.

A long-acting biodegradable contraceptive that promises to avoid some of the undesirable side-effects of medroxyprogesterone acetate is now ready for human clinical trials but will probably not be available for use in the United States for some 5–8 years. The injection of timed-release microcapsules of norethindrone enables maintenance of a constant minimal effective dose for ovulation suppression, which can continue for a month to a year or more depending on the number of microcapsules injected.

The steady low concentrations of norethindrone may not provide the menstrual dose-dependent irregularities associated with medroxyprogesterone acetate, which initially circulates at high concentrations. A phase 1 clinical trial is being launched in Mexico by investigators with a long history of clinical studies of contraception and a good record of patient compliance. Conducting initial studies outside the USA avoids delays related to FDA standards and approval.

IUD AND FUTURE DEVELOPMENTS

The IUD has grown in popularity among women throughout the world in the past decade; however, the IUD still represents only a small portion of current contraceptive practice. In 1965, less than 1% of married women used an IUD, but by 1976 more than 6% of married women and 9% of widowed, divorced, or separated women used the device. Some 10% of these women did not know what kind of IUD they were using, nor did they understand its function.

For wide application and successful use of IUDs in the future, à variety using various forms of biodegradables and polymeric delivery systems will be developed such as : (1) IUDs that will correct menstrual irregularities and certain gynecological problems; (2) IUDs for premenopausal women; (3)

IUDs for breast-feeding mothers with special nutrients for suckling babies; and (4) IUDs with nutritive elements for undernourished mothers in developing countries. It has also been proposed that some IUDs may deliver drugs to combat various communicable diseases. These new methods in IUD contraception will be developed with the help of various advances in technology, physiology, immunology, endocrinology, and biophysics - e.g. immunological concepts of blood coagulation, biophysical properties of sperm agglutination, diffusion of biodegradables, computer programming, osmotic minipumps and minianalog computers.

Computerized devices and osmotic minipumps are small, self-powered devices with continuous delivery and are implanted in some part of the body (under the arm) with no external connections. Their capabilities are constancy and precision delivery, ease of use, long-term performance, and reduction of manpower requirements. Computerized tomography, scanning electron microscopy (SEM), and X-ray dispensive microanalysis may prove useful to identify high-risk patients for certain diseases. This would then enable the physician to prescribe the most appropriate contraceptive to each individual patient.

The field of andrology (counterpart of gynecology), dealing with male reproduction, is still in its infancy compared with the knowledge accumulated thus far on female fertility and contraception. Consequently, there are not yet any widespread applications of male contraception. Comparatively, there are some major physiological differences in male and female reproductive patterns. The menstrual cycle in women lasts 28–30 days and only one or two eggs are produced per cycle. The spermatogenic cycle in man, however, is much shorter as several million sperm are produced daily.

There are also some similarities and dissimilarities between 'female menopause' and 'male andropause'. There is a reduction in the fertility of men with increasing age, but with no discrete termination. Sperm motility declines and testosterone output peaks around the age between 30 and 40 years. Libido in men is influenced by many factors other than circulating testosterone, which stimulates libido. Men between 60 and 75 years of age who maintain sexual relationships have higher testosterone concentrations than those who do not or are under institutional care.

Andropause, the decrease in sexual activity and fertility in older men, is associated with lower levels of androgen secretion by the testis and adrenal gland. There may also be a primary testicular impairment in older men. Concentrations of sex stimulating hormones may be low in some men, although the benefits of sex-hormone replacement therapy are not recommended. The spermatogenic process in man is precisely timed, and predictable periods of sterility can be induced by hormonal or pharmacological interference. Disruption of spermatogenic activity by treatment results in the absence of sperm in the ejaculate within 4–12 weeks, depending on the particular spermatogenic cells affected by treatment (cf. Cunningham *et al.,* 1980).

For biodegradables and male contraception, there are two types of compounds that can cause disruption of spermatogenesis: (1) compounds that interfere with cell division during spermatogenesis, such as colchicine and heterocyclic agents; and (2) drugs that interfere with the hormonal milieu within the testes, for example, estrogens, androgens, progestogens, and combinations of estrogen–androgen or progestogen–androgen administered in biodegradable delivery systems. All of these can interfere with the release of gonadotropins from the anterior pituitary. Antiestrogens, clomiphene citrate, and non-steroidal gonadotropin inhibitors are also effective male contraceptives.

References

Cunningham, G. R., Schill, W. B. and Hafez, E. S. E. (eds.) (1980). *Regulation of Male Fertility.* (The Hague, Netherlands: Martinus Nijhoff)

Hafez, E. S. E. (ed.) (1980). *Human Reproduction: Concentration and Contraception,* p. 509. (New York: Harper and Row)

Hafez, E. S. E. and van Os, W. A. A. (eds.) (1980a). *IUDs and Family Planning,* p. 217. (Lancaster: MTP Press)

Hafez, E. S. E. and van Os, W. A. A. (eds.) (1980b). *Biodegradables and Delivery Systems for Contraception,* p. 200. (Lancaster: MTP Press)

Hafez, E. S. E. and van Os, W. A. A. (eds.) (1980c). *IUD Pathology and Management,* p. 244. (Lancaster: MTP Press)

Potts, M. and Wood, C. (eds.) (1972). *New Concepts in Contraception,* p. 228. (Lancaster: MTP Press)

2
Morphologic features affecting IUD performance

H. M. HASSON

The quality of IUD performance is primarily dependent on the relationship of device morphology to uterine geometry. Other factors merit consideration. The incorporation of an appropriate contraceptive medication in the construction of the IUD enhances contraceptive efficacy. Variations in the biologic and socio-cultural characteristics of the wearer and in the skill and attitude of the provider influence the clinical outcome. Bernard (1971) and Mishell (1975) observed that the performance records of an individual IUD differ considerably in studies reported from different clinics and that these differences are often greater than those noted between different IUDs evaluated in the same clinic. The factors responsible for this phenomenon were collectively labelled by Mishell as the 'clinic factor'. Other authors have also identified component parts of the clinic factor (Bernard, 1971; Hasson, 1978a). The degree of skill, training, and experience of the health-care provider inserting the IUD is inversely related to the ease of use of the IUD-insertion system and method.

The elements that affect IUD performance within a given population and provider setting are related to proper device placement, size fitting, and device morphology. The importance of proper IUD placement has been documented. The device should be placed in the horizontal plane of the upper uterine segment, above the cervix and isthmus (Mann, 1962; Kamal *et al.*, 1971; Hasson *et al.*, 1976; Hasson, 1978b; Hasson, 1981).

SIGNIFICANCE OF MORPHOLOGIC IUD FEATURES RELATED TO SIZE

The size of an IUD should be fitted to the size of the host endometrial cavity. Significant disproportions between the length, width, or thickness of the IUD and the corresponding uterine parameter have been shown to be associated with increases in IUD complications (Mann, 1962; Mazher *et al.*, 1968; Tejuja and Malkani, 1969; Kamal *et al.*, 1971; Hasson *et al.*, 1976; Hasson, 1981). Presently, an IUD may be placed consistently above the level of the cervix and the size of the device selected on the basis of endometrial cavity length, by using the Wing Sound device (Hasson, 1971; Hasson, 1974b; Hasson *et al.,* 1976). This instrument measures the individual lengths of the cervical canal and the endometrial cavity, but it is not capable of predicting uterine transverse dimensions.

Although the structure of an IUD may be adapted to unknown variations in uterine transverse diameters by providing members capable of dimensional change, the degree of device adaptation is limited by geometric and mechanical constraints. To determine the longitudinal as well as the transverse dimensions of the endometrial cavity, the Wing Sound device was modified and pertinent mathematical equations were developed. The results of a recent study suggest that it is possible to obtain a two-dimensional outline of endometrial cavity shape through use of the modified instrument and method (Hasson and Dershin, 1981).

SIGNIFICANCE OF MORPHOLOGIC IUD FEATURES UNRELATED TO SIZE

Structural adaptability of the device

Morphologic IUD features, other than size, can affect IUD/uterine relationships. The structural integrity of the uterine cavity depends upon the continued existence of a favorable relation between the dimensions of the device and those of the cavity. The human uterus undergoes dynamic changes in the size and shape of its various segments during different phases of the menstrual cycle (Mann, 1962; Püroinen and Kaihola, 1975). During menstruation the isthmic segment is wide, short, and hypotonic; the fundal segment is contracted. After ovulation the activities of the two segments are reversed: the fundus relaxes, the isthmus contracts, and becomes longer and narrower (Youssef, 1958; Mann *et al.,* 1961; Mann, 1962; Johnstone *et al.,* 1974). A relatively stiff IUD with a fairly fixed shape and dimensions may have a favorable relation to its host endometrial cavity during one phase of the menstrual cycle but not during another phase (Figure 2.1). The unfavorable IUD-uterine relation may lead to clinical complications – expulsion, bleeding, infection, perforations, and pain. The IUD should be

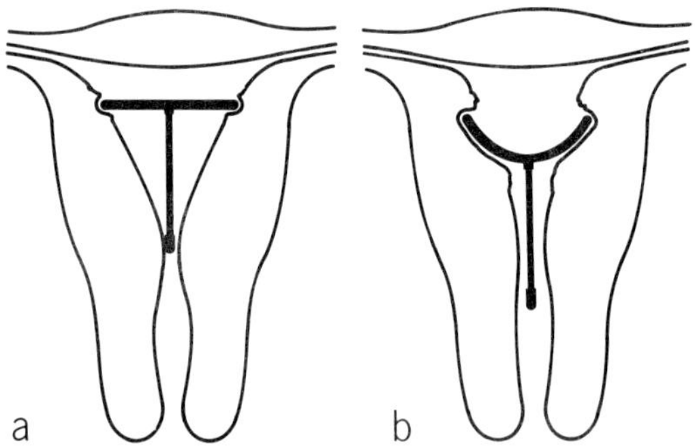

Figure 2.1 a. The Copper T: IUD–uterine relations on cycle day number 18. b. The Copper T: IUD–uterine relations on cycle day number 1

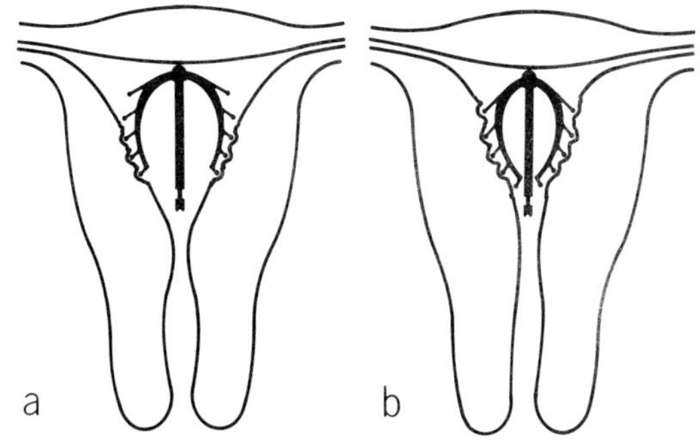

Figure 2.2 a. The Multiload: IUD–uterine relations on cycle day number 18. b. The Multiload: IUD–uterine relations on cycle day number 1

capable of undergoing adaptive structural changes in utero in response to the dynamic cyclic changes that occur in uterine shape (Figure 2.2). The adaptive IUD changes may be achieved through proper compliance properties and/or specific morphologic features.

Contour of the device

The contour of an IUD should be formed of blunt atraumatic surfaces and gentle curves (Figure 2.3a), rather than sharp edges or pointed tips (Figure 2.3b). There is convincing evidence to indicate that IUDs possessing sharp or pointed morphologic features provoke uterine injuries that may result in bleeding, perforation, and pelvic infection. The transverse arms and vertical stem of T-shaped devices possess three pointed tips. Uterine perforations caused by the pointed tips of the transverse arms and by the tip of the dependent vertical stem have been documented (Landeman *et al.*, 1973; Nygren and Johansson, 1974; Khatamee and Lehfedt, 1975; Wei, 1975; Strecker and Kraus, 1976; Tatum, 1977). Guidoin *et al.* (1976) carried out an extensive SEM study on the Dalkon Shield IUD. They found that the spicular projections of the Shield commonly became embedded into the

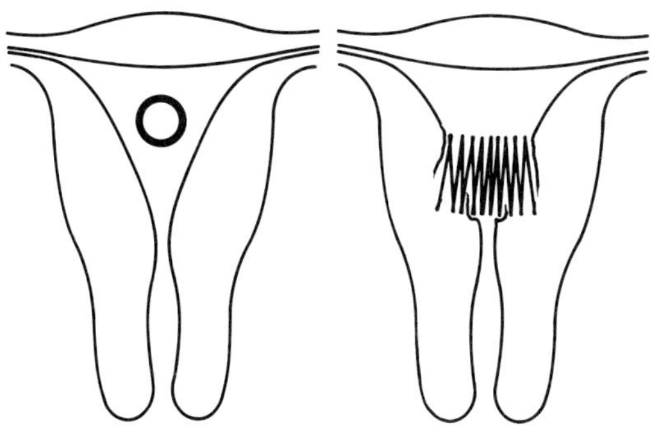

Figure 2.3 a. The Hall–Stone Ring, a device without sharp features. b. The Majzlin Spring, a device possessing sharp features

uterine wall, injuring the endometrium, and occasionally penetrated the myometrium. The uterine tissue response was one of proliferation and serious damage. An even more clear example was provided through experience with the Majzlin Spring, an IUD made of stainless-steel wire formed with 12 elbow-like projections. Women wearing the Majzlin Spring had unusually high rates of severe bleeding, pain, and infection. Of all users, 1% developed extensive pelvic cellulitis (Taylor *et al.*, 1973).

The use of IUDs that possess spicular projections is probably associated with an increased risk of pelvic infection. The pointed-device projections embed into the uterine wall within pockets containing damaged tissues. Bacteria or other organisms that manage to ascend into the genital tract through the cervix enter the uterine pockets through the endometrial ulcerations and grow in a favorable anaerobic environment.

Shape of the uppermost IUD member

The incidence of congenital uterine anomalies in patients wearing IUDs was reported to be 4% in two hysterographic studies (Adel *et al.*, 1971; Kamal *et al.*, 1971) and 9% in a third study (Mazher *et al.*, 1968). I have previously taken 150 hysterosalpingograms on patients with spontaneous abortion and found a 5% incidence of congenital uterine anomalies (Hasson, unpublished observations). These results suggest that a small but significant number of women wearing IUDs have congenital uterine anomalies, mostly of a minor type. The use of IUDs in patients with congenital fundal anomalies requires certain adaptive morphologic features. The uppermost member of the IUD must be capable of using uterine space above the tip of the fundal septum. Devices possessing such adaptive features would perform reasonably well in patients with minor uterine fundal anomalies. More marked degrees of congenital anomalies would require the use of two small IUDs or another method of contraception. Devices that do not have pertinent adaptive features are placed entirely below the tip of the fundal septum. These devices may become impacted in the lower narrow confines of the endometrial cavity and become displaced into the cervix (Mazher *et al.*, 1968; Adel *et al.*, 1971; Kamal *et al.*, 1973; Kamal *et al.*, 1975). Thus,

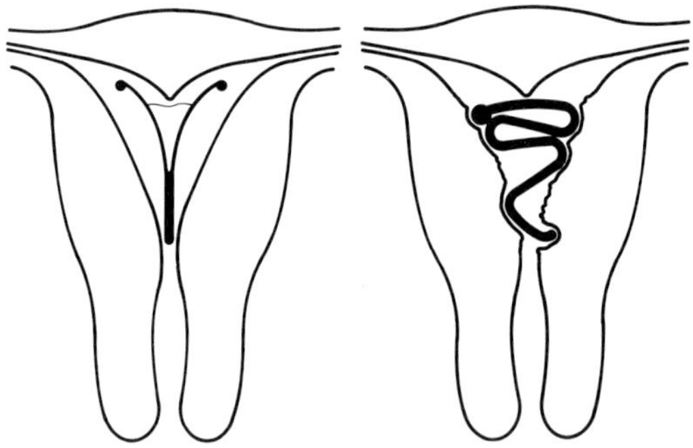

Figure 2.4 a. Position of the Ypsilon IUD within a uterus containing a small fundal septum. b. Position of the Lippes Loop IUD within a uterus containing a small fundal septum

contraceptive efficiency is decreased and the probability of expulsion, bleeding, pain, and infection is increased. Examples of IUDs with and without pertinent adaptive morphologic features are shown in Figure 2.4.

Diameter of the lowermost IUD member

Myometrial activity increases during menstruation (Behrman and Burchfield, 1968), at which time rhythmic uterine muscle contraction waves arise in the fundus and spread to the cervix (Behrman *et al.*, 1969). Uterine fundal hypertonia coexists with isthmic hypotonia; the transverse diameter of the fundus is reduced while that of the isthmus is increased. These physiologic alterations create optimal conditions for IUD expulsion during menstruation. For the IUD to remain stable in its initial high position of placement, it should have adaptive features that resist descent of the device into the lower uterine segment at the time of menses (Mann, 1962). Expanding the diameter of the lowermost IUD member is one suitable option. The enlarged lower end abuts on the uterine walls and restrains downward gravitation of the device (Figure 2.5a). IUDs possessing small lower-end diameters tend to descend into the uterine isthmus or cervix under the stress of uterine contractions, particularly when downward IUD movement is not restrained at a higher level (Figure 2.5b). Generally, devices with a small lower end have higher expulsion rates than those with a greater lower-end diameter.

Davis and Lesinski (1970) studied two devices molded in the shape of a shield. One of the devices had a tapered lower end and the other did not. The expulsion rate of the tapered device was 16%, that of the non-tapered device was 2%. Tietze (1970) evaluated first-year net expulsion rates of four IUDs. The expulsion rates were significantly higher for devices with a small lower-end diameter as compared with devices with a more expanded lower end. The expulsion rate of the copper-T IUD was found to be almost twice that of the Dalkon Shield and three times that of the Lippes Loop in more recent studies (Spellacy *et al.*, 1975; Roy *et al.*, 1976). When used

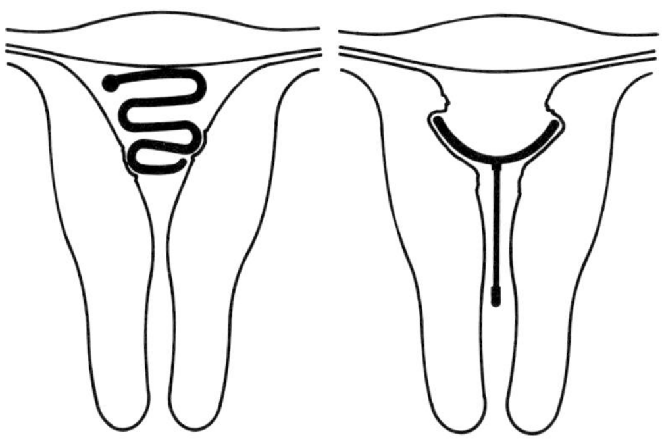

Figure 2.5 a. Uterine position of the Lippes Loop IUD after insertion: the expanded lower end restrains downward gravitation of the device. b. Uterine position of the Copper-T IUD after following insertion: the pointed lower end does not restrain downward gravitation of the device.

universally, properly constructed IUDs that are fitted to the size of the endometrial cavity are expected to yield a better record of performance than improperly constructed IUDs that are fitted at random.

References

Adel, S. K., Ghoneim, M. A. and Sobrero, A. J. (1971). Hyste:ography study of long-term effects of intrauterine contraceptive devices. *Fertil. Steril.*, **22**, 652

Behrman, S. J. and Burchfield, W. (1968). The intrauterine contraceptive device and myometrial activity. *Am. J. Obstet. Gynecol.*, **100**, 194

Behrman, S. J., Archie, J. T. and O'Brien, O. P. (1969). Myometrial activity and the IUCD. II. Propagation waves. *Am. J. Obstet. Gynecol.*, **104**, 123

Bernard, R. P. (1971). Factors governing IUD performance. *Am. J. Public Health*, **61**, 559

Davis, H. J. and Lesinski, J. (1970). Mechanism of action of intra-uterine contraceptives in women. *Obstet. Gynecol.*, **36**, 350

Guidoin, R., Courtney, J. M., Brault, R., *et al.* (1976). Intra-uterine devices. A SEM study on the Dalkon Shield. *Biomater. Med. Devices Artif. Organs*, **4**, 8

Hasson, H. M. (1971). The Wing Sound: A new uterine measuring device. *Obstet. Gynecol.*, **37**, 915

Hasson, H. M. (1974a). Differential uterine measurements recorded *in vivo*. *Obstet. Gynecol.*, **43**, 400

Hasson, H. M. (1974b). Clinical applications of the Wing Sound device. *Obstet. Gynecol.*, **43**, 498

Hasson, H. M., Berger, G. S. and Edelman, D. A. (1976). Factors affecting IUD performance. I. Endometrial cavity length. *Am. J. Obstet. Gynecol.*, **126**, 973

Hasson, H. M. (1978a). Copper IUDs. *J. Reprod. Med.*, **20**, 139

Hasson, H. M. (1978b). Factors that affect IUD performance: A review and recommendations. *J. Reprod. Med.*, **21**, 137

Hasson, H. M. (1981). Uterine geometry and IUD performance. In Hafez, E. S. E. and van Os, W. A. A. (eds.) *Medicated IUDs, Physiological and Clinical Aspects.* (The Hague: Martinus Nijhoff) (In press)

Hasson, H. M. and Dershin, H. (1981). Assessment of uterine shape by geometric means. *Contracept. Deliv. Syst.*, **2**, 59

Johnstone, F D., Boyd, I. E., McArthy, T. G., *et al.* (1974). The diameter of the uterine isthmus during the menstrual cycle, pregnancy and the puerperium. *J. Obstet. Gynaecol. Br. Commonw.*, **81**, 558

Kamal, I., Hefnawi, F., Ghoneim, M., *et al.* (1971). Dimensional and architectural disproportion between the intrauterine device and the uterine cavity. A cause of bleeding. *Fertil. Steril.*, **22**, 514

Kamal, I., Ghoneim, M., Talaat, M., *et al.* (1973). The anchoring mechanism of retention of the Copper T device. *Fertil. Steril.*, **24**, 165

Kamal, I., Ghoneim, M., Talaat, M., *et al.* (1975). Retention and expulsion of IUDs. In Hefnawi, F. and Segal, S. J. (eds.) (1975). *Analysis of Intrauterine Contraception*, p. 359. (Amsterdam: North Holland)

Khatamee, M. A. and Lehfedt, H. (1975). Hysterographic studies in women wearing Copper T devices. *Adv. Planned Parenthood*, **10**, 90

Landeman, R., Kay, R. and Wilson, K. (1973). A two man experience with the Copper T intrauterine device. *Contraception*, **7**, 477

Mann, E. C. (1962). Cineradiographic observations on intra-uterine contraceptive devices. In Tietz, C. and Leivit, S. (eds.) *Intra-Uterine Contraceptive Devices*, Series No. 54, p. 91. (Amsterdam: Excerpta Medica, International Congress

Mann, E. C., McLarn, W. D. and Hayt, D. B. (1961). The physiology and clinical significance of the uterine isthmus. Part I: The two-stage intrauterine balloon in the diagnosis and treatment of cervical incompetence. *Am. J. Obstet. Gynecol.*, **81**, 209

Mazher, K., Kamal, I. and Hefnawi, F. *et al.* (1968). A simple technic of hysterography for evaluating side effects and mode of action of intrauterine devices. *Fertil. Steril.*, **18**, 353

Mishell, D. R. (1975). The clinic factor in evaluating IUDs. In Hefnawi, F. and Segal, S. (eds.) *Analysis of Intrauterine Contraception*, p. 27. (Amsterdam: North Holland)

Nygren, K. G. and Johansson, E. P. B. (1974). Retrograde cervical perforation by the Copper T device. *Acta Obstet. Gynecol. Scand.*, **53**, 383

Püroinen, O. and Kaihola, H. L. (1975). Uterine size measured by ultrasound during the menstrual cycle. *Acta Obstet. Gynecol. Scand.*, **54**, 247

Roy, S., Azen, S. P., Mishell, D. R., *et al.* (1976). Experience with the Copper T and silicone shell loop in parous women: a randomized study. *Contraception*, **13**, 365

Spellacy, W. N., Brik, S. A. and Gordon, L. (1975). Comparative randomized study of the Copper T 200 and Dalkon Shield intrauterine devices. *Contraception*, **12**, 453

Strecker, J. R. and Kraus, H. (1976). Unusual uterine perforation by the Copper T intra-uterine device and removal by laparoscopy. *Contraception*, **13**, 47

Tatum, H. J. (1977). Clinical aspects of intrauterine contraception: circumspection 1976. *Fertil. Steril.*, **28**, 3

Taylor, W. W., Martin, F. G., Pritchard, S. A., *et al.* (1973). Complications from Majzlin Spring intrauterine device. *Obstet. Gynecol.*, **41**, 404

Tejuja, S. and Malkani, P. K. (1969). Clinical significance of correlation between size of uterine cavity and IUD. A study by planimeter-hystogram technique. *Am. J. Obstet. Gynecol.*, **105**, 620

Tietze, C. (1970). Evaluation of intrauterine devices: ninth progress report. Cooperating statistical program. *Stud. Fam. Plann.*, **55**, 1

Wei, P. Y. (1975). Downward displacement of IUDs and related problems of accidental pregnancy and cervical penetration. In Hefani, F. and Segal, S. J. (eds.) *Analysis of Intra-uterine Contraception*, p. 367. (Amsterdam: North Holland Publishing)

Youssef, A. F. (1958). The uterine isthmus and its sphincteric mechanism, a radiographic study. I. The uterine isthmus under normal conditions. *Am. J. Obstet. Gynecol.*, **75**, 1305

3
Performance of inert IUDs

L. G. KEITH AND G. S. BERGER

GENERAL COMMENTS

This chapter considers the general performance of inert devices and the factors which affect it. Both American and international data have been reviewed.

IUDs are an accepted method of family planning throughout the world. Millions of women in developing and developed countries depend on IUDs to prevent unwanted pregnancy (Huber *et al.*, 1975). Despite certain known adverse side-effects (Edelman *et al.*, 1979), IUDs are considered a relatively safe and effective method of family planning by health-care professionals and governmental regulatory agencies (US Departments of Health, Education, and Welfare, 1968, 1978).

One of the major advantages of the IUD is its high continuation rate. Depending upon the medical circumstances in which an IUD is inserted (i.e. interval, postpartum or post-abortion) and selected patient characteristics (i.e. age, parity, social class, and cultural background), as many as 75% of women receiving an IUD continue to use it for at least 1 year (US Departments of Health, Education, and Welfare 1978; Tietze and Lewit, 1970). Unlike the oral contraceptives or vaginal barrier methods, discontinuation of an IUD requires a positive action on the part of the patient and/or the clinician who is providing her care.

After the reintroduction of IUDs into the clinical practice of medicine in 1959, dozens of devices have been designed and tested (Table 3.1). Of these, a far smaller number have come to market. Devices generally have been classified as inert or medicated. Inert devices most commonly are made of a plastic polymer, while medicated devices incorporate some additional antifertility agent such as a metal (copper) or hormone (progesterone). These agents act to enhance device effectiveness and reduce the incidence of IUD-associated pregnancies.

Table 3.1 IUDs that have been evaluated[a]

Ahmed	Hall–Stone Ring	Quadracoil
Ammeo IUD	Heart	Ragab Ring
Anchor	Hulka	Robinson
Antigon	Icon	Russian Cross
Beospir	Intrauterine Pleated Membrane	Saf-T-Coil
Birnberg Bow	K. S. Wing	Shamrock
Butterfly	Latex Leaf	Silent Protector
China Ring	Lem	Soonawalla Y
Coralle	Lippes Loop	Spira Ring
Cuivre	Louvred Device	Spiran W
Cu-T	M	Spring Coil
Cu-7 (Gravigard)	Marko	Szontagh
Dana	Majzlin Spring	TR-10
Dalkon Shield	Margulies Spiral (Gynecoil)	U-Coil
DIU Pharmatex	Massouras Duck's Foot	Winata
FD-1	Monterrey	Ypsilon
Flower of Canton	Multiload	Yusei Ring
Fluid Filled Tecna	Omega	Zazil Delta A
Ghorbani	Ota Ring	Zipper Ring
Gräfenberg Ring	Progestasert	

[a] From Edelman *et al.*, 1979

EVALUATION OF IUD PERFORMANCE

After 20 years of clinical usage, there is no completely satisfactory way to measure the efficacy of IUDs. Before the recognition of the utility of the life table method of analysis (Tietze and Lewit, 1973), the effectiveness of IUDs often was reported in terms of events per 100 woman-years of IUD use. This statistic, commonly known as the Pearl Index, was computed from the formula:

$$\frac{\text{Number of events}}{\text{Total woman-months of IUD use}} \times 1200$$

The problem with the Pearl Index is that it cannot account for the time when events occur. Since women discontinue using their IUDs at different post-insertional times and for different reasons, the life table method was found to be a more effective analytic tool because it could be used to compute the probability of occurrence of IUD-related events as a function of time from IUD insertion (Tietze and Lewit, 1973). A simplified explanation of this method has been presented elsewhere (Edelman *et al.*, 1979):

'The two basic assumptions which underlie use of the life table method are: (1) the risks of terminating IUD use for any reason may depend on the length of time since IUD insertion, but are the same for all women at any time interval from IUD insertion; and (2) women who are lost to follow-up have essentially the same IUD experience as women who are not lost to follow-up.

'The basic data required for the computation of life table rates include:

(1) the duration of IUD use from the insertion for each continuing IUD user, (2) the duration of IUD use from insertion to discontinuation for all women who have withdrawn from observation, and (3) the reasons for withdrawal (e.g. pregnancy, expulsion, removal, lost from further observation). Time is usually measured in months, but any unit of time may be used. The data are then used to calculate net or gross life table rates for each type of IUD event. These rates are computed for each unit of time and as a cumulative rate over time.

'The difference between net and gross life table rates is illustrated in terms of pregnancy rates. The net pregnancy rate is calculated on the basis that women may leave the study for reasons other than pregnancy, such as expulsion or removal, before they have had a chance to become pregnant. On the other hand, the gross pregnancy rate provides an estimate of the pregnancy rate as if pregnancy were the only reason for withdrawal from observation. Both net and gross rates give event probabilities per woman, or rates per 100 women, and can be computed for any duration of IUD use. The net rates for all possible termination reasons add up exactly to the total termination rate for all reasons combined. Net rates are used to report the experience of a group of women using one type of IUD. Gross rates should be used for the comparison of specific events for two or more IUDs or groups of women.'

Mode of action of IUDs

From the patient's point of view, the question of how the IUD works may be more important than once thought (Tatum, 1979). This question is particularly relevant in terms of subsequent fertility which may be adversely affected if the patient develops a clinical infection with the IUD *in situ*. If infection occurs, it often is difficult, if not impossible, to determine whether or not the IUD was causally related to the infection or whether the patient's life style, sexual preferences, and exposure to venereal diseases were at fault (Edelman *et al.*, 1979).

Subsequent complications notwithstanding, it is clear that the antifertility effect of non-medicated IUDs in humans originates promptly in the uterus, disappears quickly, is not negated by menstruation, and does not interfere with the normal estrogen–progesterone balance (Tatum, 1979). Despite much detailed study in the past two decades, the exact mode(s) of action of IUDs remain(s) unknown. Animal research has been extensive, but the conclusions to date have been difficult to extrapolate to humans because of extensive species variations (Keith *et al.*, 1978). The single observation common to all species is the IUD's ability to evoke a local inflammatory response in the endometrium. This local response in some way probably sets up a train of events which is anticonceptional in nature. Whether or not this local response is the precursor of later, more generalized inflammatory responses in those patients who subsequently develop clinical signs and symptoms of pelvic infection is not clear.

Logically speaking, there are four biological events which may be vulnerable to the action of IUDs: (1) inhibition or interference with ovulation; (2) interference with fertilization; (3) interference with blastocyst implantation; and (4) early destruction (abortion) of the implanted blastocyst.

Because of the known failures of the IUD which result in intrauterine or extrauterine pregnancies, it is unlikely that the first event takes place to any extent. A similar statement may be made with regard to interference with fertilization. It is more likely that some interplay with the blastocyst takes place and that this activity forms the basis of the successful activity of the IUD.

The presence of an IUD may additionally influence coital activity, a factor which also may affect fertility. This is of particular importance in those cultures which proscribe intercourse when the woman is bleeding.

Detailed discussions of the possible mechanism(s) of action of the IUD have been presented elsewhere (Edelman *et al.*, 1979; US Departments of Health, Education, and Welfare, 1978; Tatum, 1979). In addition, the potential role of prostaglandins in this process has been described extensively (Toppozada and Hafez, 1979).

Method of study of IUD performance

Since the inception of the Cooperative Statistical Program (CSP) of the Population Council under the direction of Christopher Tietze in 1963, it has become accepted practice to report IUD performance in terms of net annual rates of pregnancy, expulsion, and removal per 100 women. The use of this methodology has the distinct advantage in that it permits comparisons at given points in time (e.g. 12, 24, 36 and 48 months) between different IUDs or different studies with the same device.

A somewhat different approach has been suggested recently on the basis of the three epidemiologic considerations which are part of any evaluation of IUD performance: (1) the agent (IUD); (2) the host (woman); and (3) the environment surrounding the insertion (the clinician) (Chi *et al.*, 1978). While this concept appears attractive, it is difficult to obtain adequate comparative data from the literature on all aspects of each epidemiologic factor, as older studies do not invariably address them. Nonetheless, the following discussion will utilize these broad major headings and interrelate them to the life-table method where possible.

THE AGENT

Geometric parameters

As early as 1974, it was observed that there was a direct correlation between IUD surface area and IUD effectiveness (Andolsek, 1974). This observation subsequently was confirmed by other workers (Davis and Lesinski, 1970; Ragab, 1973; Wheeler *et al.*, 1974). As the IUD surface area increases, so does its effectiveness. Increases in IUD surface area are also accompanied by increases in removal rates for pain and bleeding, so that the benefit of size is negated to some extent by the problem of side-effects. These relationships are illustrated in Figure 3.1.

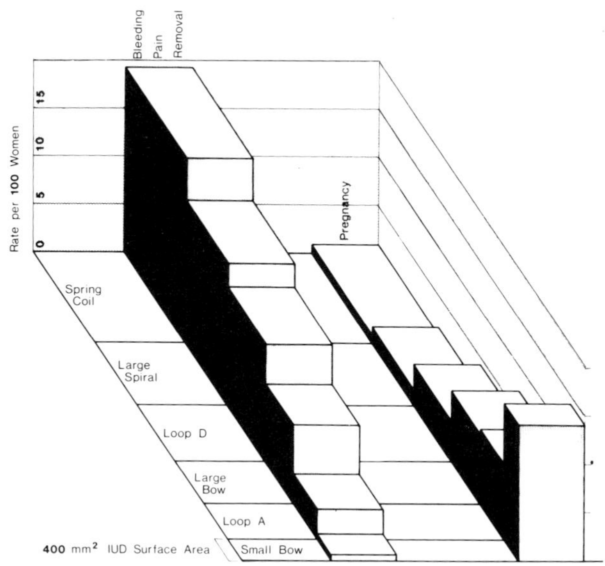

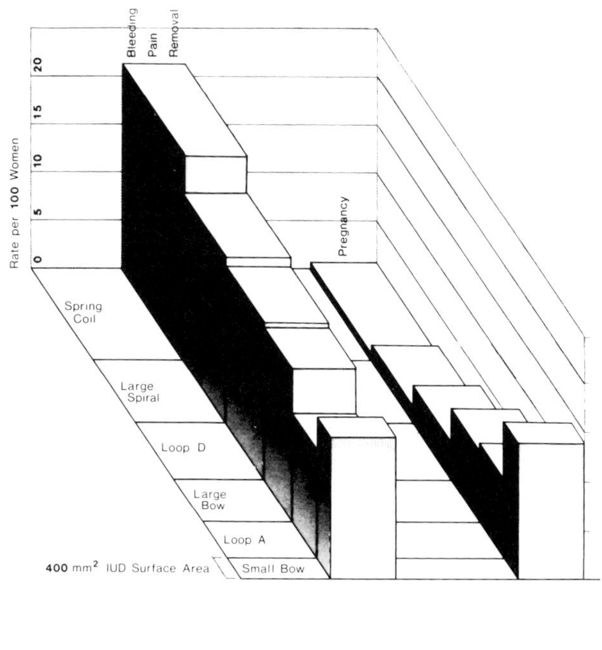

Figure 3.1 a. Two-year pregnancy and bleeding/pain removal rates for selected inert IUDs as a function of their surface area (From Andolsek, 1974). b. Two-year pregnancy and bleeding/pain removal rates for selected IUDs (From Bernstine *et al.*, 1975)

It is presently unclear whether surface area acts alone or in association with other spatial factors such as thickness, volume, and size, all of which may change with changes in surface area. Most observations relating to the geometry of IUDs have been made on linear devices. It cannot be stated with certainty if they apply directly to membrane or shield devices, although recent work points in this direction (Hasson and Sharrett, 1980). Table 3.2 presents comparison of the geometric parameters of many inert IUDs.

Table 3.2 Geometric parameters of inert IUDs[a]

IUD	*Size*[b] (mm)	*Thickness* (mm)	*Surface area* (cm^2)	*Volume* (cm^3)
Loop	15.5	2.50	10.2	0.6
Loop D	17.5	2.64	13.7	0.7
M-213	20.0	2.50	2.47	0.1
Majzlin Spring	22.5	2.51	4.58	0.1
Gräfenberg Ring	12	2.16	9.16	0.2
Saf-T-Coil	22.5	2.93	8.07	0.5
Birnberg Bow	18	2.26	9.22	0.5
Ota Ring	12.5	2.50	12.1	0.2
Ypsilon	31	2.70	21.1	0.4
Antigon-F	15	2.85	11.4	0.5
Dalkon Shield	14	1.47	12.66	0.3

[a] From Bernstine *et al.*, 1975
[b] Smallest circumscribing circle

Other considerations

Beside those factors relating to the geometry of the device (configuration, size, surface area, thickness, and consistency), there are three other 'agent' factors which may relate to performance. They are type of inserter, type of packaging, and the presence or absence of medication.

In particular, the width of the inserter is of crucial importance. A thick, rigid inserter has the disadvantage of possible insertional difficulties in nulliparas or in patients with acute ante- or retropositional changes. On the other hand, a thin, malleable inserter lends itself to use in these groups of patients. While some clinicians routinely administer a paracervical block before insertion of an IUD, this by no means is universally practiced.

Two major constraints impinge on the design of the inserter: (1) the need to avoid perforation; and (2) the need to achieve a high fundal placement to insure maximum efficacy and retention with minimal side-effects (Bernstine *et al.*, 1975). There are two basic types of inserters: the stick type and the tube-and-rod type. The former often is notched in one or more places to hold the IUD; the inserter used with the Dalkon Shield is an example. The latter is used more often today because it permits a device to be momentarily stretched into a linear configuration at the time of insertion and to regain its original shape quickly after uterine placement (e.g. Lippes Loop, Double Spiral). Tubular inserters are generally more flexible than stick inserters. This flexibility allows the clinician to preshape the inserter in the direction of the uterine axis as determined by sounding. The tube-and-rod type inserter probably presents the optimum configuration to avoid trauma and permit a correct fundal placement. The absence of trauma at the time of insertion can be viewed only as a positive sign by the patient and one which does not discourage her continued use of the IUD. For the clinician, correct fundal placement is essential for effectiveness.

With regard to packaging, those packages which require the presence of an assistant to maintain sterility deter IUD use. Conversely, any package which permits a no-glove, no-touch, sterile insertional technique allows a broad use of the IUD in a variety of clinical settings.

The IUD tail

The presence of the tail on the IUD may or may not affect performance. Clearly, the tail is of value in facilitating easy removal of the IUD without the need to probe inside the uterine cavity with a hook device. On the other hand, the tail often represents a source of discomfort to the partner or source of irritation to the patient if it is left too long.

The tail question received international attention at the time of the Dalkon Shield controversy in 1974. The tails of some of the Dalkon Shields were composed of many microfilaments encased in a nylon sheath (Tatum *et al.*, 1975). In contrast, most other IUDs studied at that time had monofilament tails. It was suggested that the multifilament tails led to a 'wicking effect' (Tatum *et al.*, 1975). Because of the implications which followed the presentation of these findings, most authorities now insist that tails be of a monofilament nature. To our knowledge, the work on the 'wicking'effect has never been duplicated in the published literature. In any event, it is unlikely that the presence of a tail contributes directly to IUD performance in prevention of pregnancy.

Spatial relations

Major advances in knowledge of the spatial relationship of the IUD have taken place in recent years (Hasson *et al.*, 1976). Before that, it had been shown that the incidence of IUD-associated bleeding and pain probably was related to the disparity between the size of the uterus and the IUD (Tejuja and Malkani, 1969). Device efficacy (expressed in terms of event rates for pregnancy, expulsion, and removal for pain and bleeding) has been correlated with the closeness of the match between the IUD size and that of the uterine cavity (Hasson *et al.*, 1976). The best IUD performance occurred when the IUD was about 1.5 cm shorter than the true uterine cavity length as measured by the Wing Sound. The worst performance occurred either when the device length exceeded the cavity length or when it was 2 or more cm shorter than the cavity. In these situations, event rates approached or exceeded 50%. The implication of both of these studies is that better results could be obtained if IUDs were selectively fitted to each woman (Hasson, 1974). Sufficient data pertaining to prescription fitting of IUDs do not yet exist.

THE HOST

Age and parity

Both age and parity influence IUD performance as measured by standard rates of pregnancy, expulsion, and removal for bleeding and pain. In an evaluation of these two factors as they related to inert IUDs (Lippes D), the pregnancy rate declined as the age of the patient increased (Bernstine *et al.*, 1975). Similarly, the pregnancy rate declined as parity increased. The expulsion rate also declined with age and parity, with age the more important factor (Bernstine *et al.*, 1975). Removals for medical reasons decreased more with increasing parity than with increasing age (Bernstine *et al.*, 1975). When the Lippes D is considered, the 2-year continuation rate per 100 women was 58 for ages 15–24 and 75.4 for ages 35–39 (Bernstine *et al.*, 1975). Patients who were para 1 or 2 had a 2-year continuation rate of 59.5 with the Lippes Loop D, whereas patients with parity of 5 or more demonstrated a 2-year continuation rate of 74.1.

Time of insertion

The IUD can be inserted at any time during the menstrual cycle, including immediately after abortion or term delivery. What is not clear is if there is a truly preferable time. In the past, many clinicians were reluctant to insert IUDs after delivery or abortion because they feared increased likelihood of perforation. Others have been reluctant to perform interval insertions when the patient was not menstruating for fear of disturbing an intact, early pregnancy.

Notwithstanding the personal preferences of the clinician, the most important clinical concern is a significantly higher expulsion rate after post-partum insertions (Bernstine *et al.*, 1975; Edelman *et al.*, 1979). On the other hand, IUDs inserted after first-trimester abortion are generally not associated with significant differences in event rates when compared with interval insertions (Edelman *et al.*, 1979).

Uterine size and position

As mentioned above, there is a relationship between uterine size, device size, and device performance. It is not common clinical practice to accurately measure uterine dimensions *perse* before IUD insertion, although this can be done with the Wing Sound device (Hasson, 1974; Hasson and Dershin, 1981). Even if this capability exists, it is doubted that its application will be widespread except in the hands of the most sophisticated clinicians. With accurate intrauterine dimensional measurements, many of the problems leading to pregnancy, expulsion, or removal can be eliminated or at least markedly reduced, irrespective of the device selected. The clinician who wishes to select an IUD size based on dimensional uterine measurements may find that this single factor is of great importance in minimizing adverse event rates.

Few existing reports on IUDs attempt to correlate event rates with uterine position. For the Lippes D, retroversion is associated with lower pregnancy, expulsion, and removal rates at 1 year (Chi *et al.,* 1978). Interestingly, pregnancy and medical removals with another non-medicated device (the Dalkon Shield) were slightly higher (Chi *et al.,* 1978).

The significance of these observations is debatable, because the finding of severe anteversion or retroversion may present a considerable technical obstacle to insertion in the hands of some clinicians. Unless the insertion is performed in a manner by which the uterus is maximally straightened by traction on the cervical tenaculum and bending the device to the shape of the cavity, insertion may be into the lower uterine segment. This in itself may predispose to pregnancy, expulsion, or symptoms leading to medical removal.

Socio-cultural factors

A variety of socio-cultural factors influence the woman and her ability to tolerate the IUD. Among them are her education, place of residence, religion, economic status, desire for future children, prior contraceptive history, and the availability of alternative methods of birth control. Within a given social setting, one or more of these may attain prominence.

For example, in those societies which proscribe intercourse during the times that a woman is bleeding, spotting or prolonged menses may become so objectionable as to lead to a request by the husband for removal of the device, even though the patient remains happy and unconcerned. Similarly, women who are less well educated may be less understanding of some of the side-effects of IUDs as well as some of the precautions required for their continued safe use. At the same time, living in an urban setting may mean easier access to medical facilities and better chance to evaluate side-effects which may result in IUD removal.

These findings are of interest, but at present we are unable to state with certainty that socio-cultural factors are of greater or lesser overall importance than are those factors related to the device *per se* in any overall evaluation of IUD performance.

Other considerations

The association between IUD use and pelvic infection has been discussed extensively. Of the numerous comments which have been published in the last 5 years, three will be mentioned here because they underscore the difficulty in making any definitive statements which can be considered as guidelines for future planning with regard to IUD use.

The degree of polymorpholeukocytic infiltration is greater in the excised tubes of women undergoing sterilization while wearing an IUD than in the tubes of a similar group of women who undergo sterilization while not wearing an IUD (Smith and Soderstrom, 1976). The implication of this finding is that the presence of IUD in the uterus may affect the 'background' level of inflammatory response in the tubes. It is important to recognize, however, that these patients were *totally asymptomatic* whether or not they were using an IUD at the time of their surgical sterilization. Moreover, those with IUDs had no more postoperative infection than those who had no IUDs (Smith and Soderstrom, 1976).

Repeated episodes of 'PID' in IUD users are more likely to lead to subsequent sterility (Westrom *et al.,* 1976). This observation has important implications for women whether or not they are using an IUD. It recognizes, in a tangential manner, what has been apparent to many clinicians for years; that is, that certain patients apparently are 'PID prone'. In some of these women, the multiplicity and choice of partners may play a part in their recurrent infections, but it is clear that not all PID is gonococcal in origin. It is precisely because the clinician so often is unable to wait for bacteriological confirmation before instituting therapy that the diagnosis and treatment of PID is often on an empirical basis.

The long-term prognosis for women with repeated episodes of PID will depend to a great extent on whether an early initial episode takes one of three courses: (1) resolved, (2) indolent, or (3) acute catastrophic course (Figure 3.2).

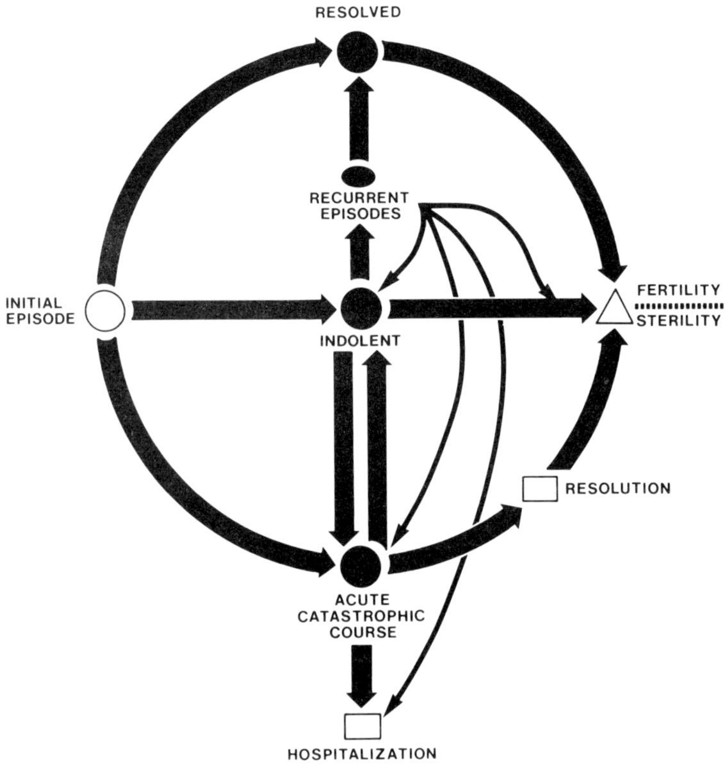

Figure 3.2 Possible progression of PID

The complexity of the problem is seen clearly. Many authorities are concerned that post-PID sterility will affect large numbers of women. Should these women require surgical correction for their conditions, the cost of modern microsurgical repair even of simple clubbed tubes will be prohibitive for the average woman (Keith and Berger, 1981).

The frequently quoted statement that the use of an IUD is associated with a 3–5 times greater risk of PID may have had an effect on IUD utilization in the United States. Although there is no national family planning program with comprehensive statistical information available for review, the data available from the private and public sectors document a slow but continuing decline in IUD use by American women in the past few years (Keith and Berger, 1980). How much of this decline is directly due to patient concern regarding infection cannot be stated. There is evidence, however, that the incidence of PID within a population fluctuates over time and between geographic locations, depending on a variety of social as well as medical situations. Since the IUD wearer is sexually active, she is exposed to a variable but definite risk of PID which is independent of her IUD use. A more detailed discussion of the relation of PID to IUD use has been provided elsewhere (Edelman *et al.*, 1980).

THE CLINIC (CLINICIAN)

Of the factors which influence the performance of IUDs (i.e., the agent, the host, and the environment in which the IUD is inserted), the latter has received far less attention than either of the former. To be sure, scattered reports document a variety of clinic-related circumstances which supposedly affect IUD performance. Unfortunately, no consistent pattern exists from country to country for all devices or from clinic to clinic for a given device (Keith *et al.*, 1978; Chi *et al.*, 1978). In our opinion, three aspects of the clinical setting are worthy of mention because of their general applicability to the broad question of IUD performance.

Physical location of the clinic

Whether the clinic is in an urban or rural setting may be crucial to its ability to attract well-trained staff members. This statement applies equally to physicians, nurses, counselors, etc. It is likely, but not always the case, that urban clinics present a more attractive and intellectually stimulating work setting for health professionals. In addition, the urban clinic's case load may be large enough to require institution of specialized 'mini-clinics' in which all patients seen at a given time receive the same type of service (i.e., family planning). The rural clinic, on the other hand, may be forced to mix patients desiring family planning services with a variety of other patients, some of whom may be ill or require great and urgent attention. In such circumstances, the family planning patient may get less than optimal care. Furthermore, the attitudes of medical personnel in rural areas are sometimes less open toward family planning than those of their urban counterparts. Should this indeed be the case, the individual practitioner may have little motivation either to acquire or to improve on those skills requisite for successful IUD insertion and follow-up.

Within a given country, all clinics undoubtedly are influenced by the general policy of the Government toward family planning and the IUD in particular. In a country such as the United States, where there is no national family planning program, IUD use has declined gradually in the past few years (Keith and Berger, 1981). This has occurred not so much because the governmental health regulatory agencies have spoken against the IUD but rather because they never strongly favored it. The lack of clear-cut pro-IUD statements became obvious when the IUD was receiving great amounts of adverse attention from the popular media. Other countries, on the other hand, have run successful IUD programs as part of organized family planning service at the national level. Their results, in terms of averted pregnancies, avoided abortions, and prolonged continuation rates, have been well documented (Huber *et al.,* 1975).

Experience of the clinician

When IUDs first were reintroduced into medical practice, there was little question that physicians were interested in adding them to the existing contraceptive armamentarium. Perhaps because the uterus was invaded, the medical community believed that IUD insertion was a task best performed by physicians. Often, however, scant attention was given to training physicians how to perform insertions properly. As a result, many physicians learned by the 'see one, do one, teach one' technique and soon became disenchanted with their results. Apart from this, the basic concept that IUDs required physicians for insertion was soon challenged on several points (Ostergard and Marshall, 1974). The debate which ensued has not yet been settled (Manisoff and Tyrer, 1980).

In the United States, well-trained nurses and paramedics indeed have equally good or better performance records with IUDs than physicians whose training often was presumed to be part and parcel of their medical degree (Ostergard and Marshall, 1974). The crux of the argument lay in the training itself. The nurses went to class, learned the technique, were taught on mannequins, and were supervised for their early work. The successful results of these early physician expander programs undoubtedly became the forerunner of the now popular Family Planning Nurse Practitioner Courses, some of which last as long as 4 months on a full-time basis. The acceptance of trained Family Planning Nurse Practitioners was enhanced by a liberal attitude from Planned Parenthood of America (Manisoff and Tyrer, 1980). The use of Family Planning Nurses to insert IUDs is spreading to other public agencies and also to the private sector of medicine.

Many countries which have national family planning programs recognized that they could never be successful if they relied solely on physicians to serve all patients desiring family planning services. In these circumstances, midwives, nurses, and, in some cases, talented lay persons were pressed into service. It became clear that with training all these individuals could insert IUDs in a manner similar to physicians and thus release the physician to do more specialized tasks.

Over the years, the performance of these non-physician clinicians has been reported from a variety of different geographic, cultural, medical, and social settings. Variations have been observed in IUD performance, related complications, continuation rates, and preferences for specific types of IUDs.

Follow-up

No discussion of IUD performance can be complete without a thorough consideration of follow-up. It clearly must be understood that unless the clinician knows what has happened to the patient in whom an IUD has been inserted, any other information on that patient (the host), the IUD (the agent), and the environment may fall into the category of accumulated data from which little can be learned. While we do not propose a universal follow-up system, we believe that for any system to work there are five requisites if large numbers of patients are to be seen:

(1) It must be well thought out in advance.
(2) The clinician must consciously decide what outcome variables will be considered.
(3) The system should allow for those variables, but be flexible enough to delete or add information as required.
(4) If interclinic, interdevice comparisons are to be made some thought should be given to selecting variables which lend themselves to such comparisons.
(5) If large numbers of patients are to be followed up the facilities of a data-retrieval system are essential.

It is particularly important that any follow-up program avoid the temptation to gather too much information. Such systems become so data heavy that they are unresponsive to change. A good follow-up system should monitor the quality of care provided and assist the clinician in recognizing the problems as they arise. Such systems need not be elaborate nor expensive, and can be designed specifically to fit local needs.

CONCLUDING REMARKS

Even though the exact mechanism of action of IUDs is presently unclear, the single observation common to all IUDs is their ability to evoke a local inflammatory response in the endometrium. Among the device-related factors which affect IUD performance are the following: (1) geometric parameters; (2) type and size of inserter; and (3) type of packaging. It is presently unclear whether the tail affects IUD performance.

The woman using the IUD affects its performance in relation to: (1) her age and parity; (2) the time of the insertion; (3) the size and position of the uterus; and (4) a variety of socio-cultural factors. The presence or absence of a history of PID may be an important determinant of IUD performance and acceptance.

Not as well understood are some of the clinical factors which affect IUD performance: (1) physical location of the clinic (rural and urban); (2)

qualifications of the clinician; and (3) follow-up. All are essential in evaluating IUD performance.

Acknowledgment

Supported in part by the Charles A. Fields Medical Foundation and The Center For The Advancement Of Reproductive Health.

References

Andolsek, L. (1974). The Ljubljana IUD experience: 10 years. In *Program Abstracts, Third International Conference of Intrauterine Contraception*, Cairo, Egypt, p. 17

Bernstine, R. L., Davidson, A. R., Duncan, G. W., Kalkward, D. R., Sikov, M. R., Wheeler, R. G., and Williford, J. F. (1975). Review and analysis of the scientific and clinical data on the safety, efficacy, adverse reactions, biological action, utilization, and design of intrauterine devices. (Washington, D.C.; US Department of Commerce, National Technical Information Service, PB-249 614)

Chi, I., Kessel, E. and Mitra, M. (1978). An epidemiologic study of intrauterine contraceptive devices: A preliminary report. In Sciarra, J. J., Zatuchni, G. and Speidel, J. (eds.), *Risks, Benefits and Controversies in Fertility Control*, p. 478. (Hagerstown, Md.: Harper and Row)

Davis, H. J., and Lesinski, J. (1970). Mechanism of IUDs in women. *Obstet. Gynecol.*, **36**, 350

Edelman, D., Berger G. S. and Keith, L. (1979). *Intrauterine Devices and Their Complications*. (Boston, Ma.: G. K. Hall & Company)

Edelman, D. A., Berger, G. S. and Keith L. G. (1980). Major complications of intrauterine devices. In Keith, L. G., Kent, D. R., Berger, G. S. and Brittain, J. R. (eds.) *The Safety of Fertility Control*, p. 131 (New York: Springer)

Hasson, H. M. (1974). Clinical applications of the Wing Sound device. *Obstet. Gynecol.*, **43**, 498

Hasson, H. M., Berger, G. S. and Edelman, D. A. (1976). Factors affecting intrauterine contraceptive device performance. I. Endometrial cavity length. *Am. J. Obstet. Gynecol.*, **126**, 973

Hasson, H. M. and Dershin, H. (1981). Assessment of uterine shape by geometric means. *Contracept. Deliv. Syst.*, **2**, 59

Hasson, H. M. and Sharrett, S. A. (1980). Selective fitting of IUDs. *Scientific Exhibit, Twenty-eighth annual Clinical Meeting, The American College of Obstetricians and Gynecologists*, New Orleans, La., May 3–8

Huber, S. C., Piotrow, P. T. and Orlans, F. B. (1975). Intrauterine devices. In: *Population Reports*, Series B, No. 2, p. 48. (Washington, D.C.: University Medical Center)

Keith, L. G. and Berger, G. S. (1980). IUDs and family planning in the United States. In Hafez, E. S. E. (ed.) *Progress in Contraceptive Delivery Systems*, Vol. 2, p. 83. (Lancaster: MTP Press)

Keith, L. and Berger, G. S. (1981). Optimal utilization of the microsurgeon. In Phillips, J. J., (ed.) *Microsurgery II*. (Downey, Ca.: American Association of Gynecologic Laparoscopists) (In press)

Keith, L., Hughey, M. and Berger, G. S. (1978). Experience with modern inert IUDs to date: A review and comments. *J. Reprod. Med.*, **20**, 125

Manisoff, M. and Tyrer, L. B. (1980). The nurse practitioner's role in family planning. In Keith, L. G., Kent, D. R., Berger, G. S. and Brittain, J. R. (eds.) *The Safety of Fertility Control*, p. 27. (New York: Springer Publishing)

Ostergard, D. R. and Marshall, J. R. (1974). The training of nurse-midwives in family planning at Downstate Medical Center. In Morehead J. E. (ed.) *Paramedical Personnel in Family Planning – A Creative Partnership* (Boston, Md.: The Pathfinder Fund)

Ragab, M. I. (1973). IUDs on trial. In Hasegawa, T., Hayashi, M., Ebling, F. J., *et al.* (eds.) *Proceedings of the Fertility and Sterility Conference*, International Congress Series, No. 278, p. 958. (New York: Excerpta Medica Foundation)

Smith, M. R. and Soderstrom, R. (1976). Salpingitis: A frequent response to intrauterine contraception. *J. Reprod. Med.*, **16**, 159

Tatum, H. (1979). Clinical aspects of intrauterine contraception: Circumspection 1976. In Wallach, E. and Kempers R. (eds.) *Modern Trends in Infertility and Conception Control*, p. 333. (Baltimore, Md.: Williams and Wilkins)

Tatum, H., Schmidt, F., Phillips, D., McCarty, M. and O'Leary, W. (1975). The Dalkon Shield controversy: Structural and bacteriologic studies of IUD tails. *J.Am. Med. Assoc.*, **231**, 711.

Tejuja, S. and Malkani, P. K. (1969). Clinical significance of correlation between size of uterine cavity and IUCD: A study by planimeter-hysterogram technique. *Am. J. Obstet. Gynecol.*, **105**, 620.

Tietze, C. and Lewit, S. (1970). Evaluation of IUDs: Ninth progress report of the Cooperative Statistical Program. *Stud. Fam. Planning*, **55**, 1

Tietze, C. and Lewit, S. (1973). Recommended procedures for the statistical evaluation of intrauterine contraception. *Stud. Fam. Planning*, **4**, 35

Toppozada, M. and Hafez, E. S. E. (1979). The role of prostaglandins in the mechanism of action and side-effects of IUDs. In Hafez, E. S. E. and van Os, W. A. A. (eds.) *Medicated IUDs and Polymeric Delivery Systems, Book of Abstracts*, No. 23. Proceedings International Symposium, Amsterdam, Holland, June 27–30

US Departments of Health, Education and Welfare, Food and Drug Administration, Advisory Committee on Obstetrics and Gynecology (1968). *Report on Intrauterine Contraceptive Devices*. (Washington, D.C.: US Government Printing Office)

US Departments of Health, Education and Welfare, Food and Drug Administration, The Medical Device and Drug Advisory Committees on Obstetrics and Gynecology (1978). *Second Report on Intrauterine Contraceptive Devices*. (Washington, D.C.: US Government Printing Office)

Westrom, L., Bengstsson, L. P. and March, P. A. (1976). The risk of pelvic inflammatory disease in women using intrauterine contraceptive devices as compared to non-users. *Lancet*, **2**, 221

Wheeler, R. G. Duncan, G. W. and Speidel, J. J. (1974). *Intrauterine Device-Development, Evaluation and Implementation*, pp. 107, 245. (New York: Academic Press)

4
Development of copper IUDs

J. ZIPPER

Medicated endouterine contraception was studied after a series of basic findings that prompted development of this concept and its extension to clinical use after a critical evaluation of non-medicated endouterine contraception (in use since the beginning of the century). From these studies, the Cu-7 and Cu-T IUDs were developed and are presently in extended clinical use. In the late 1950s, interest in this new, yet old, technology was renewed. In 1962, research began in the rat and rabbit (Zipper *et al.* 1969a), where the effects of an endouterine foreign body in these species was noted. Marked differences were demonstrated in the physiological behavior of the rat and rabbit after implanting an endouterine foreign body. The most relevant finding was perhaps the generalized anti-implantation action in the rat uteri in the presence of a small foreign body; while in the rabbit, the foreign body caused a local action that permitted implantation in other areas of the same uterus.

RELEVANT FINDINGS OF EARLY STUDIES

In the rabbit these were that normal implantation never occurred in the uterine area occupied by the thread; that blastocysts were able to implant under and over the area occupied by the thread; that the number of corpus lutea present in both ovaries did not differ significantly ($p < 0.5$); and that the basic mechanism affected was implantation.

In the rat, no implantation occurred in the uterus bearing the thread, irrespective of its size. Elimination of the thread in the second day post-coitus permitted implantation of the blastocyst after a normal process of fertilization. The number of corpus lutea present in the ovary of the treated side was significantly less than in the control ($p < 0.01$). Estral rhythm was significantly altered in the treated animals, estrus often persisting for 48 hours. A massive leukocyte infiltration was found in the treated uterus, and the basic mechanism affected was implantation. The differences in physiological behavior of these two species led to using the rabbit as the experimental species. By using a number of metabolic inhibitors of the reproductive process by a system of slow release in a small area of the uterine cavity, their effects as contraceptive agents were observed. Alterations of implantation must be attributed to the influence of the pharmacologic agents used, and not to the foreign body.

Research was first oriented to the action of pure metallic cations introduced into the uterus in the form of very thin wires (Zipper *et al.*, 1969a). The effect of copper, zinc, silver, tin, and magnesium on implantation rates in rabbits was studied by introducing a wire of each of these metals separately into the inferior portion of one uterus near the cervical os. The depressive effect on implantation rates in the uterus treated with copper and zinc was demonstrated. Silver, tin, or magnesium did not induce this effect. Specific histological changes were produced in the endometrium by copper (estrogenic endometrium) and silver (progestative endometrium). The possibility of using the effects produced by different oligoelements as a contraceptive technique was also discussed. The histological effect observed led us to study the effects of endometrial hormonal receptors in this and other species, and to begin the development of medicated contraception in man (Zipper *et al.*, 1963; Zipper and Medel, 1974; Zipper *et al.*, 1969b).

The smallest quantities of zinc or copper required to block the enzymatic system sensitive to these metals were unknown, as were the actions of either sperm or blastocysts on this system. The endometrium was one target of these cations. Copper did not have a systemic effect on other systems, because a contralateral uterus and ovary behaved normally. The importance of the catalytic contraceptive effect of copper lay in its low toxicity and in the possibility of a controlled and slow liberation from a wire. This concept of contraception through metallic oligoelements added a new dimension to the contraceptive mechanisms of a non-medicated IUD (Zipper *et al.*, 1969b).

PHYSIOLOGICAL BASIS FOR THE USE OF METALLIC TRACE ELEMENTS AS LOCAL CONTRACEPTIVE AGENTS

Metallic trace elements are essential constituents of all living systems and are usually present in only extremely small quantities compared with the organic components. They may be present in as low a ratio as one atom to a million, this ratio usually being sufficient for the normal continuance of biological processes. Metals within cells generally function as biologic catalysts and are associated with a protein as a prosthetic group or are alone without being directly linked to a protein. When alone they may be able to displace or neutralize the trace metals in a metal–enzyme complex. Through this mechanism, the rate of biological reactions may be altered. The metal ions can also be linked to metal buffers, since the reaction of a metal ion with a nucleophilic partner is one form of neutralization.

The copper ion is probably one of the most versatile catalysts of all metals and participates in a great variety of physiologic reactions. Copper is a member of the first transition series of elements, which share common properties; most are present as essential trace elements in biologic systems.

This series comprises the elements with atomic numbers 21–30: scandium, titanium, vanadium, chromium, magnesium, iron, cobalt, nickel, copper, and zinc. Because of their chemical similarities, the last two elements – copper and zinc – are highly specific antagonists. Copper is one of the most reactive of all elements in this series. It is capable of reacting with a variety of amino acids and proteins more strongly than most metal ions. The metal exists in three states: as a neutral atom, a cuprous ion, and a cupric ion. It may be oxidized directly by atmospheric oxygen and the copper-containing enzymes are essential in the metabolic oxidation cycle. Copper is also capable of oxidizing a large number of chemical groups, such as phenyl- , sulfhydryl- , amino- , etc. It can also participate in trans-sulf-hydration and hydrolysis.

METAL-ION ANTAGONISM

Nearly all metal ions of the periodic table can activate or inactivate some enzymatic systems. In the case of copper-containing enzymes, two metals – molybdenum and zinc – play a significant role *in vivo*. An excess of molybdenum exerts a profound effect on copper enzymes which can be counteracted specifically by additional copper. An excess of zinc in the rat produces anemia due to the displacement of copper, iron, and cobalt, resulting in a corresponding deficiency of these three trace elements. Anemia produced by a zinc excess can be reversed by supplementing copper, iron, or cobalt. Ordinarily, when the concentration of copper in liver is increased, that of zinc in the same organ is reduced.

KNOWN PHYSIOLOGICAL MECHANISMS THAT REGULATE THE CONCENTRATION OF COPPER AND OTHER RELATED TRACE ELEMENTS

Normal copper concentration in the human endometrium averages from 14.5 μg/g protein in the early proliferative phase to 16.6 μg/g protein in the late secretory phase. These figures are significantly different ($p \langle 0.001$). Zinc concentration increases from 206.3 to 325.0 μg/g over the same time ($p \langle 0.001$) (Hagenfeld, 1972).

Plasma and hepatic copper are regulated by the hormones of the pituitary–adrenal system. Both values are increased after hypophysectomy or adrenalectomy.

Experiments performed in monkeys indicate that low doses of copper (1 mg/kg body weight), stimulate caeruloplasmin synthesis while higher doses depress it. Estrogenic and progestational action have been investigated in relation to copper metabolism.

The phenomenon of plasma copper concentration increase during pregnancy has been known since 1928. In 1961, zinc concentrations were found to be lowered in this physiological state. This is also found in women taking oral contraceptive pills. Experimental studies in rat indicate that the estrogenic compound – mestranol – causes a reduction in plasma zinc concentration. Norethindrome, the progestational compound, does not produce this alteration. Zinc uptake is increased in the liver, spleen, adrenals, and uterus in rats treated with mestranol.

The importance of the role of ovarian hormone (estrogen and progesterone) in the metabolism of plasma and tissue copper and zinc suggests that the excess of some of these metals might play a role in the normal physiology of the target organ of these hormones. In all animal species studied thus far, the presence of copper cations in the uterine cavity produced marked effects on fertility. Even highly toxic metals produce less contraceptive effectiveness than copper, suggesting that the effect produced by this metal is highly specific. Studies performed to determine the concentration and variation of certain trace elements in the normal human endometrium during the menstrual cycle demonstrated that zinc concentration is increased in the late secretory period, and that copper concentration is increased throughout the secretory period. Manganese concentration is very high in the early proliferation phase, exceeding that of all the other phases, and sodium and potassium cations are in a higher concentration in the proliferative than in the secretory periods.

Copper and zinc cation concentrations in the endometrium, cervical mucus, and serum in women using copper IUDs for 1 year can be summarized as follows. Endometrial copper concentration was increased during the time the Cu-T was *in situ* 2–3 times the normal amount. (Hagenfeld and Landgren, 1975). Copper can be detected through histochemical techniques only in the secretory period (Salaverry *et al.,* 1973).

METALS AND SEX STEROIDS

Cadmium interferes with the tropic effect of estrogen in the uterus of ovariectomized rats. The stimulating action of testosterone propionate on male accessory sex organs is inhibited by a variety of metals, including copper. However, molybdenum salts can selectively enhance the androgenic action of testosterone propionate in castrated animals. Topical applications of cadmium or copper to one of the uterine horns of a rat prevents implantation for an extended period, without affecting ovulation, which indicates a metal-dependent mechanism associated with steroids at the molecular level.

METALS AND THE NERVOUS SYSTEM

An intravenous infection of copper salts induces ovulation in the rabbit and frog. In the rat, an electrolytic deposition of copper in the preoptic region of the hypothalamus induces ovulation, although the specific biochemical steps activated by the metal in the hypothalamic region are unknown.

THE MALE REPRODUCTIVE SYSTEM

Zinc is the most abundant of the metals associated with the functions of the male reproductive system. Considerable quantities of zinc are found in the prostatic gland, epididymis, testes, seminal fluid, and spermatozoa. This high concentration is not directly related to the concentration of zinc-containing enzymes.

Zinc deficiencies in normal animals usually result in degeneration and atrophy of the testes, as well as in hypoplasia of the coagulating glands and the seminal vesicles. With the exception of testicular atrophy, all these changes can be reversed by the administration of zinc. In experimental animals or in man, primary endocrine manifestations of zinc deficiency in both sexes are consistent with hypopituitarism.

Testis

The deleterious effect of many trace elements has been tested. The action of subcutaneously administered copper sulfate was also studied. In contrast to cadmium, where the seminiferous tubules are completely destroyed with a single injection, copper arrests spermatogenesis, causes almost complete degeneration of epididymal spermatozoa, and produces slight necrosis of the head of the epididymis. Alteration of the epididymis is the most constant finding with copper and, in contrast to cadmium, the histophysiological alterations produced are reversible.

Spermatozoa

Copper and zinc are normal constituents of humal seminal plasma and spermatozoa. Any imbalance of these ions can be lethal for the spermatozoa. The marked toxicity of copper salts in sperm was described for the first time in 1853. In 1948, the importance of sulfhydryl groups for the motility and metabolism of sperm was established. Sperm motility and fructolysis can be inhibited *in vitro* by very low concentrations of copper ions. These effects of copper can be counteracted by SH-compounds such as cysteine, glutathione and ergothionein, a sulfhydryl-containing base which is a natural constituent of seminal plasma.

THE FEMALE REPRODUCTIVE SYSTEM

In the female reproductive tract, one of the most important protein enzymes, for which zinc is a cofactor, is carbonic anhydrase. In the rabbit, this enzyme is directly associated with the progestative response of the endometrium. In the non-pregnant, or non-progestational, endometrium in general, this enzyme is almost absent in most species. In sheep, however, carbonic anhydrase is equally active in the non-pregnant and pregnancy states. In the rat there is carbonic anhydrase activity in the decidua. This enzyme is similary characteristic of the placenta, specifically in the maternal portion. In the female rat, experimentally produced zinc deficiency does not have an irreversible effect on the reproductive system during pregnancy, although gross malformation is produced in the fetus.

Uterine motility

Endouterine copper or zinc has a marked effect on uterine motility in the rabbit (Medel *et al.*, 1974). Copper and zinc wires sutured to the uterine cavity with absorbable catgut or inserted free into the lumen were maintained inside the uterus for prolonged periods, whereas segments of polyethylene were expelled as soon as they were released from the uterine wall by dissolution of the anchoring suture. *In vitro* uterine motility increases as copper salt concentration rises in the milieu. Zinc salts have the inverse effect.

To summarize, copper and zinc, when placed in the uterine cavity, produce alterations in the uterine physiology of the species studied, leading to a marked decrease in fertility of the uterine horn containing the intrauterine metallic device. Antifertility effects are local and relate to alteration of the endometrial milieu.

THE ROLE OF COPPER IN THE DEVELOPMENT OF IMPROVED IUDs

Extensive clinical studies have attempted to prove that non-medicated IUDs are no longer as promising as once was thought. It is even questionable whether any of the newer plastic devices have given any better continuation rates than the original Grafenberg device.

Removals for medical reasons - pregnancies and expulsions - were dependent on the physical properties of the inert material used. The size, surface area, and stiffness were essentially of utmost importance. A device with a larger surface area would always offer a lower pregnancy rate and a higher removal rate, because metrorrhagia and pain from all devices were directly related to the surface area. If stiffness was increased, expulsion decreased but metrorrhagia increased. The physical and biological properties required to obtain an optimum contraceptive result, with low metrorrhagia and low expulsion rates, were intrinsically opposed. Because of these limitations, non-medicated IUDs have failed to give continuation rates significantly different from each other.

Correlation of the physical characteristics on related clinical manifestations through which clinical efficiency of a non-medicated device can be predicted are as follows:

(1) The rate of accidental pregnancy is inversely related to the endometrial surface covered by the device in the area of normal implantation.

(2) The occurrence of metrorrhagia and/or pain directly relates to the area of the endometrium in contact with the device, and to the pressure which the device exerts upon the myometrium.

(3) The rate of first expulsion is inversely proportional to the stiffness of the device where retention is governed primarily by the resilience of the device (Zipper *et al.*, 1970, 1972, 1973, 1975).

These deficiencies of non-medicated IUDs led to the formulation of a new system of intrauterine contraception. This method depended on an antifertility material that could act locally on the uterine cavity, added to a carrier, which in itself would minimally disturb the uterus. A number of agents were considered that could inhibit fertility when used locally, such as pharmacological agents, hormones, and metals. Trace metals were considered of greatest interest. Of these, animal studies showed that metallic copper had the highest activity and, in the form of an IUD, could provide a reservoir for prolonged effectiveness.

Intrauterine contraception is equivalent in concept to topical therapy for other parts of the body, such as the skin or the eyes, where the desired therapeutical effect (in this case, fertility control) is accomplished by applying maximum drug concentration locally to the site of treatment, with a minimum possibility of affecting secondary structures.

Despite these obvious benefits in patient acceptability, clinical experience showed that this contraceptive system, using metallic copper, could be improved. The T-shaped device (the carrier) has a cross-sectional diameter that, when folded for insertion into the uterus, sometimes made introduction through the cervix difficult. This situation was not uncommon in nulliparous women, a group in whom local intrauterine contraception was particularly indicated. This led to the development of the '7'-shaped carrier which, when folded, was at least 30% smaller in diameter than the 'T'.

Clinical contraceptive effectiveness has been extensively analyzed in two copper-carrying IUDs: the Cu-T and the Cu-7, with comparable plastic composition and surface, to which copper wire was wound to the vertical arm (Zipper *et al.*, 1973). By increasing the copper surface, the pregnancy rate decreases. These devices were also tested according to the location of copper on the device (Zipper *et al.*, 1973).

Contraceptive effectiveness of intrauterine copper added to a vector has an optimal value at 200 mm^2 of copper. Expulsion rates for a given vector change in relation to the copper surface and to the location of the metal inside the uterus. A minimum expulsion rate was observed when copper was located in the medial–vertical region of the uterine cavity. As copper approaches the implantation area, expulsion rates increase, suggesting a change of the uterine motility pattern. When copper is wound on the vertical arm, the optimum surface area to minimize expulsion is 120 mm^2 of copper. Copper and zinc have a clear effect on uterine motility: copper activates whereas zinc inhibits (Zipper *et al.*, 1970 Medel *et al.*, 1972, 1976).

With the Cu-7 IUD, pregnancy and removal rates are not significantly different from those obtained with the Cu-T-200 IUD; neither are continuation rates. This is due to similarity in the relation between surface of the device, metallic surface, and location of copper in the uterine cavity, plus the stiffness of the carriers as they differ only in shape. The Cu-7 IUD also offers certain advantages in this regard, since its introduction diameter, when folded, is more reduced and specially suited for nulligravides.

The rate of metrorrhagia does not increase when the amount of copper is increased. This is of fundamental importance, since the pharmacologically active level can easily be increased without producing bleeding, which is the essential limiting factor of intrauterine non-medicated devices.

The most important clinical problem that leads to discontinuation of use is irregular menstrual bleeding. This is produced by the plastic vector rather than by the added copper (Zipper *et al.*, 1977a).

DURABILITY OF ENDOUTERINE COPPER

The quantitative analysis of devices with 200 mm^2 of copper, made with a 0.2 mm diameter wire and exposed to the uterine milieu for up to 480 days, indicated a daily dissolution of approximately 40 μg with a tendency to gradually decrease. The average corrosion rate is 14.5 ± 5.3 mg/year, 69 ± 20 μg/day per device with an average dosage of 55 ± 18 μg/day per device. A linear extrapolation leads to the prediction of 50% penetration in 3 years. This assumption is conservative regarding real penetration rates since the rate decreases with time of use.

Contraceptive effectiveness of the Cu-7 and Cu-T-200 has not altered in its fourth year of use (Zipper *et al.*, 1974) (Tables 4.1 and 4.2). Removal of the device after 48 months of use, and the gravimetric quantifications of the copper wire, indicated an average of 68 mg of remaining copper, while the average weight of the wire was initially 95 mg. There must be a loss in the progressive loss of copper, starting in the second year of use, since the initial calculations indicated a loss of approximately 18.5 mg in the first year. The Cu-7-200 with a 0.2 mm diameter wire will presumably offer a duration of more than 5 years. A slight increase in the copper wire will produce a device of more than 10 years' active life.

ELECTROCHEMICAL EFFECTS OF INTRAUTERINE METALS

The introduction of metal inside the uterine cavity creates an electrochemical effect measuring electrical potentials in copper IUD users alone, and others that form an electric pair CuZn (copper upper portion of the uterus) and ZnCu (copper lower portion) (Zipper *et al.*, 1976a).

Endouterine potential before the introduction of the metallic device, measured with non-polarizable electrodes, was positive at the fundus with respect of the uterus. The placement of dissimilar metal electrodes in the uterus induces voltage gradients that are roughly predictable from the metals' cell potential in blood as electrolytes. When copper and zinc electrodes are placed at opposite ends in the uterus, they induce voltage gradients that are typically higher than 100 mV/cm. External copper and zinc wires connected at one end, and with the other ends in contact with various positions on the skin, alter gradient potentials in the uterus.

When a length of zinc wire was wound around the upper portion of the stem of a small Cu-7-200, it took about 1 year after insertion for the zinc to disappear. When the zinc wire was wound around the lower portion of the stem, it disappeared in 1 month. Zinc reduced copper intrauterine corrosion; this was more effective when zinc was located in the lower portion. Since corrosion is far below the standard Cu-7 copper loss, it seems that zinc in the inferior portion completely suppresses copper corrosion as long as it lasts. There is also some residual copper protection even after the zinc is gone.

The role of zinc added to a copper IUD in improving contraceptive efficacy has been established. Preliminary evidence indicated that the placement of the zinc, hence the polarity of the IUD, influences expulsion rates. According to *in vitro* and animal studies, the motility of uterine smooth muscles varies inversely with the concentration of copper ions. The effects of IUD polarity on IUD expulsion have not been separated experimentally from copper ion concentration effects. Larger and more definitive studies will be required to ascertain the effect of voltage gradients in the uterus on

Table 4.1 Net cumulative rates of events per 100 users of Cu-7-200 IUD, by type of termination[a]

	12 months			24 months			36 months			48 months		
Type of termination	*Rate*	*LL*[b]	*UL*[b]	*Rate*	*LL*	*UL*	*Rate*	*LL*	*UL*	*Rate*	*LL*	*UL*
Pregnancy	2	0.9	4	4	2	6	5	3	8	6	4	8
Expulsion	5	3	7	5	3	7	5	3	7	6	4	8
Removals:												
Bleeding/pain	2	0.7	3	3	2	5	5	3	7	5	3	7
Other medical	1			2			2			2		
Personal reasons	0.8			2			3			3		
Planning pregnancy	3			9			15			20		
Total termination	13			26			35			42		
Continuation rate	87			74			65			58		
Woman-months of use		55 530			9862			12 918			15 243	

[a] After 516 initial insertions
[b] 95% confidence limits are shown for pregnancy, expulsions, and bleeding/pain: LL = lower limit; UL = upper limit

Table 4.2 Net annual rates of events per 100 users of Cu-7-200 IUD, by type of termination[a]

Type of termination	1 year			2 years			3 years			4 years		
	Rate	*LL*	*UL*	*Rate*	*LL*	*UL*	*Rate*	*LL*	*UL*	*Rate*	*LL*	*UL*
Pregnancy	3	0.9	4	2	0.7	4	2	0.8	5	0.9	0.1	3
Expulsion	5	3	76	0.8	0.2	2	0.7	0.0	1	0.4	0.0	3
Removals:												
Bleeding/pain	2	0.7	3	2	0.9	4	1	3	3	0.9	0.1	3
Other medical	1	0.5	3	0.8	0.2	2	0.7	3	3	0.0	0.0	2
Other personal	0.8	0.2	2	1	0.4	3	0.8	3	3	0.9	0.1	3
Planningpregnancy	3	1	4	8	5	11	7	10	10	8	4	12
Total termination	13.3	10.2	16.4	14.6	10.9	18.1	11.6	7.7	15.4	11.0	6.8	15.2
Continuations	86.7			85.4			88.4			89.0		
Woman-months of use		5553			4309.5			3055.5			2320.5	
No. of women beginning each year		516			404			299			228	

[a] 95% confidence limits given: LL = lower limit; UL = upper limit

IUD event rates, and to separate ion copper effects *per se* from electrolytic effects. (Zipper *et al.*, 1976b, 1977a,b).

MECHANISM OF ACTION OF ENDOUTERINE COPPER

Non-medicated IUDs

The mechanisms of action of non-medicated IUDs differ in the various studied species. In man, as well as in rodents, an intrauterine foreign body produces an outpouring of acute and chronic inflammatory cells into the uterine fluid and the produce of their cytolysis was toxic to the blastocyst, preventing implantation. This no longer seems relevant in primates or in man, since in severely polymorph-depleted rats induced with rabbit antisera to rat neutrophils, the IUD works adequately. The inflammatory process plays a minimal role, if any, in the mechanism of action of the IUD. Although there is no uniform agreement as to the mechanism of action of non-medicated IUDs, the following may partially explain their contraceptive mechanism and metrorrhagic action: (1) alteration in endogenous steroidal metabolism; (2) an accelerated production of uterine prostaglandins that would induce an anticipated menstrual period; and (3) the fibrinolytic activity induced by IUDs.

Medicated IUDs

Most experiments investigating the mechanism of copper have attempted to dissociate the action of the vector from that of the pharmacologic agent. The modifications of the endometrium differ in the proliferative and secretory phases and relate to changes in the concentration of the different cations, enzymes, and steroidal receptors of the mucosa. There is a decrease in the number of sperm that reach the fallopian tubes of copper IUD users, compared with women with plastic devices or those using no contraceptive device. Important alterations of sperm morphology have also been observed. Other demonstrated effects of endouterine copper on physiological parameters are related to tubal–uterine motility. A marked action on rat uterine motility *in vitro* has been observed as copper concentration increases, while zinc produced an intense inhibition of uterine motility *in vitro*. Other experiments show that copper induces an increase in radioactive 17β-estradiol uptake in rats (Aedo and Zipper, 1973), while it also stimulates a much greater local exudation of leukocytes than that evoked by plastic devices.

CONCLUDING REMARKS

Copper IUDs produce a marked increase in endometrial copper and a decrease in endometrial zinc in the secretory phase. The enzymes, alkaline phosphatase and β-glucuronidase, decrease in the secretory phase and acid phosphatase activity increases, but there is an inhibition of α-amylase activity. Effects on steroidal receptors can be demonstrated, but seem to be specific for each species. Kinetic studies in rabbit have demonstrated that copper is a competitive inhibitor at the receptor level, affecting the progesterone more than the estrogen receptors, which could explain the morphologic suppression of the progestational effect in this species. The greater stability of estrogen receptors in the presence of copper would also explain increased estradiol uptake in rat uteri with a copper-bearing IUD.

The physiological parameters that are modified by endouterine copper and that produce a decrease of fertility bear reference to endometrial physiology (endouterine cations, endouterine enzymes, and estrogenic receptors); ovum transport and spermatic physiology.

References

Aedo, A. R. and Zipper, J. (1973). Effect of copper intrauterine devices on estrogen and progesterone uptake by the rat uterus. *Fertil. Steril.*, **24**, 345

Hagenfeld, K. (1972). Studies on the mode of action of the Copper-T device. *Acta Endocrinol. (Suppl.) (Kbh)*, **71**, 169

Hagenfeld, K. and Landgren, B. M. (1975). Local effect of medicated IUDs. In Hefnawi, F. and Segak, S. J. (eds.) *Analysis of Intrauterine Contraception*, p. 349. (New York: Elsevier)

Medel, M., Espinoza, C., Zipper, F. and Prager, R. (1972). Reversibility of the contraceptive action of copper and zinc in the rat and rabbit. *Contraception*, **6**, 241

Medel, M., Espinoza, C., Zipper, J. and Prager, R. (1974). Preliminary observation on the effects of copper, zinc and polyethylene IUFB on the uterine motility of the rabbit. *Contraception*, **5**, 2

Medel, M., Zipper, J., Dabancens, A., Thamas, A. and Thomas, E. M. (1976). Contraceptive efficacy of two different metals using a modified seven vector. *Int. J. Gynecol. Obstet.*, **14**, 194

Salaverry, G., Mendez, M., Zipper, J. and Medel, M. (1973). Copper determination and localization in different morphologic components of human endometrium during the menstrual cycle in copper intrauterine contraceptive device wearers. *Am. J. Obstet. Gynecol.*, **115**, 163

Zipper, J. and Medel, M. (1974). Factors that limit the efficiency of copper-carrying IUDs. In Wheeler, A. B., Duncan, C. D. and Speidel, E. F. (eds.) *Intrauterine Devices.* (London: Academic Press)

Zipper, J., Delgado, H. and Guillof, E. (1963). Estudios experimentales del mecanismo de acción de cuerpos intrauterinos. *Rev. Child. Obstet. Gynecol.*, **28**, 18

Zipper, F., Medel, M. and Prager, R. (1969a). Suppression of fertility by intrauterine copper and zinc in rabbits. *Am. J. Obstet. Gynecol.*, **105**, 529

Zipper, J., Tatum, H. T., Pastene, L. and Medel, M. (1969b). Metallic copper as an intrauterine contraceptive adjunct to the 'T' device. *Am. J. Obstet. Gynecol.*, **105**, 1274.

Zipper, J., Tatum, H. J., Medel, M., Pastene, L. and Rivera, M. (1970). Human fertility control through the use of endouterine metal antagonisms of trace elements (EMATE). Presented at the *Nobel Symposium 15*, May 19–27

Zipper, J., Segura, R., Medel, M. and Torres, L. (1972). Biological action of copper. Development of a new type of intrauterine contraception-Cu7. *Aust. N. Z. J. Obstet. Gynecol.* Proc. IPPF South-East Asia & Oceania Congress, Sydney

Zipper, J., Medel, M. and Segura, R. (1973). Intrauterine Contraception. In *Proceedings of the 5th International Congress on Pharmacology*, San Francisco, 1972, vol. 1, p. 195

Zipper, J., Medel, M. and Dabancens, A. (1974). Studies on a new seven device (small seven) containing copper and copper-zinc. Contraceptive potentiation by using metallic association. (New York: Excerpta Medica International) In *Proceedings of the 1st International Congress on Human Reproduction*, Series No. 370.

Zipper, F., Medel, M., Pastene, L., Torres, L., Osorio, A., Rivera, M. and Toscanini, C. (1975). Studies of the physiological activity of IUDs containing copper. *Contraception*, **12**, 1

Zipper, J., Medel, M., Pastene, L., Rivera, M., Torres, L., Osorio, A. and Toscanini, C.

(1976a). Four year experience with the Cu-7 200 device. Endouterine copper in fertility control. *Contraception*, **13**, 7

Zipper, J., Medel, M., Osorio, A., Goldsmith, A. and Edelman, D. A. (1976b). Long-term use effectiveness of the Cu-7200 IUD. *Int. J. Gynecol. Obstet.*, **14**, 142

Zipper, J., Edelman, D. A. and Goldsmith, A. (1977a). An overview of IUD research and implications to the future. *Int. J. Gynecol. Obstet.*, **15**,

Zipper, J., Wheeler, R., Adrián, H. and Angelo, S. (1977b). Electrochemical effects of metals on IUDs. *Int. J. Fertil.*, **22**, 155

Part II
APPLICATIONS AND COMPLICATIONS OF IUDs

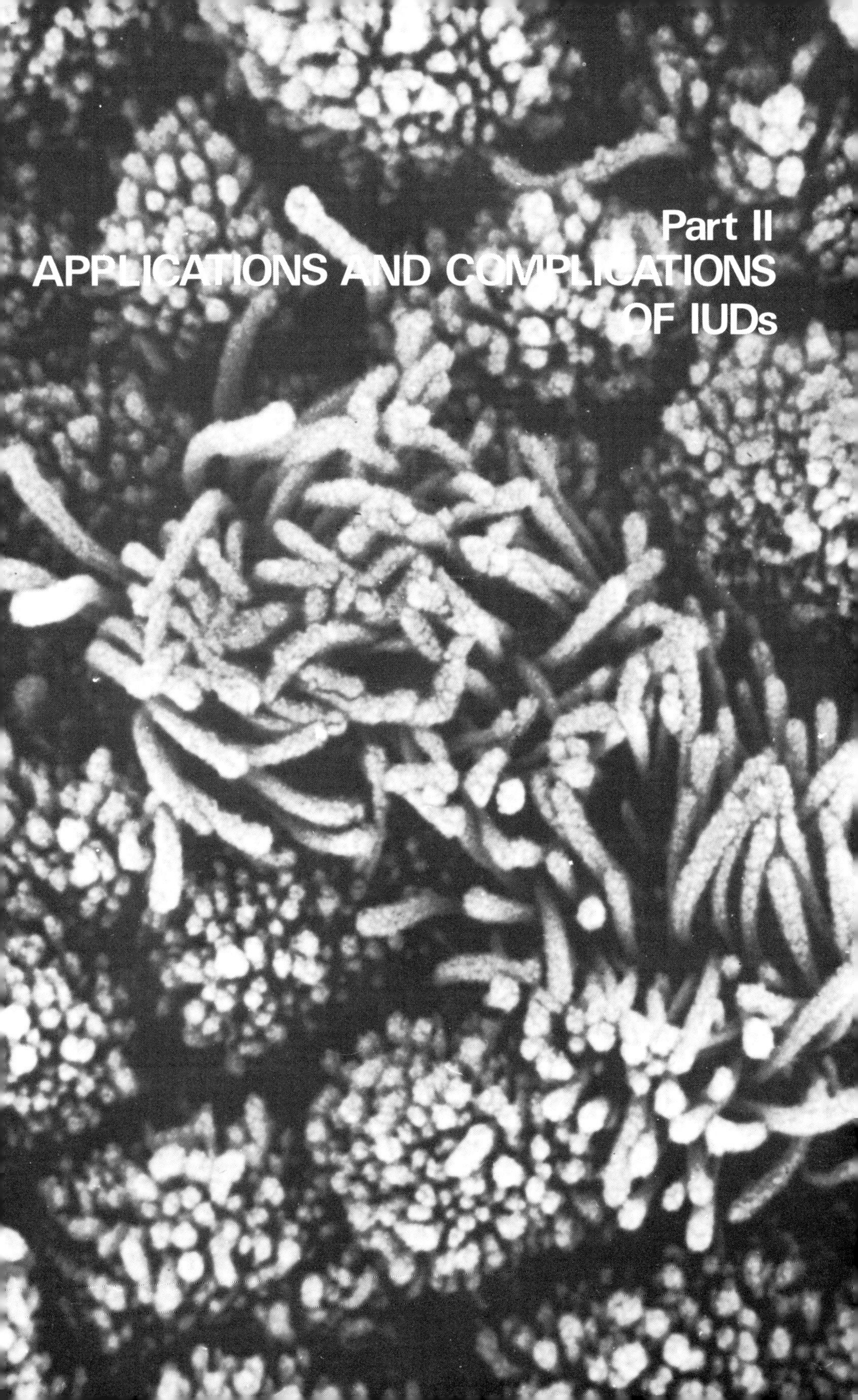

5
Contraindications, complications and methods of IUD insertion

M. F. HAYES AND K. S. MOGHISSI

The intrauterine device (IUD) is a widely used method of contraception with an acceptable failure rate of 1–6 per 100 woman-years of use. It does not require daily attention by the user, as do oral contraceptive agents. It requires no motivation or special effort before coitus, as do barrier methods. The patient for whom the IUD is indicated might be defined as the woman who desires this means of contraception and who has no contraindications.

CONTRAINDICATIONS

Pregnancy

Pregnancy is an absolute contraindication to IUD insertion. The pregnant woman may be under the erroneous impression that insertion of an IUD may cause termination of her unwanted pregnancy. What she will not know is that spontaneous abortion resulting from an IUD is associated with high morbidity and mortality. For this reason, it is imperative that a bimanual examination be performed before insertion of an IUD, and if pregnancy is suspected, a pregnancy test obtained. It is also recommended that IUDs be inserted during menstruation.

Infection

An IUD must never be inserted if there is evidence of active pelvic infection. The patient should be treated and instructed to return after her full course of antibiotics, and again in 3 months. If there is no evidence of recurrence, and if the patient does not wish for further pregnancies, an IUD may be inserted. An IUD should not be inserted in the patient with previous pelvic inflammatory disease (PID) or ectopic pregnancy who wishes to bear children. Similarly, an IUD is contraindicated with a history of recurrent PID regardless of childbearing plans. A woman with active cervicitis should be treated before IUD insertion. The patient with multiple sexual partners is at high risk of contracting pelvic infection and the use of an IUD should be avoided in this individual. Owing to the increased risk of PID and other complications, many physicians prefer not to insert IUDs in nulliparas.

Abnormalities of uterine shape

For an IUD to give maximum protection, it must be in close contact with the uterine fundus, conform to the uterine configuration, and must not be expelled. Any abnormalities which create mechanical problems preventing good position precludes IUD use. These include congenital anomalies, such as bicornuate or arcuate uterus, and uterine myomata. A very small uterus will quickly and painfully attempt to expel an IUD. Severe cervical stenosis will not allow insertion without dilatation.

Abnormal cytology

The patient whose cervicovaginal smear is abnormal requires further evaluation and treatment. If an IUD is inserted before diagnostic studies, the patient may not return, and the opportunity for early diagnosis of a serious condition may be lost.

Menstrual abnormalities

The IUD should never be used in a woman with undiagnosed menorrhagia or metrorrhagia. If these conditions are present and pathology has been ruled out or the patient has been adequately treated, the IUD may be used. The progesterone-releasing IUD (Progestasert) may be useful in such cases since it decreases uterine bleeding.

Anemia

All IUDs except the Progestasert have been shown to increase blood loss (Luukkainen and Nilsson, 1978; Rybo and Bergqvist, 1978; Zador *et al.*, 1976). This is of particular importance in developing countries, where anemia and malnutrition are common. Anemia may be considered a relative contraindication to contraception with the IUD, unless a Progestasert is available.

Coagulopathy or blood dyscrasia

Once again, these patients should use no device which will worsen their already compromised state of health.

Endometrial hyperplasia

Adenomatous hyperplasia is considered by some to be premalignant. Abnormal bleeding induced by IUD use may be difficult to differentiate from that caused by recurrent hyperplasia. If an IUD is inserted, two potential complications are added. First, any abnormal bleeding may be overlooked, being attributed to the IUD. Second, endometrial biopsy, a good method of following up these patients, may be avoided due to fear of dislodging the IUD.

Severe dysmenorrhea

The IUD may enhance dysmenorrhea, especially cramping and backache. The patient should be warned of this before insertion. The Progestasert may be a good choice for such patients.

Valvular heart disease

Any foreign body, the IUD included, is a potential source of septic emboli. The patient with valvular heart disease, already at risk for subacute bacterial endocarditis, should use another method of contraception.

Abnormal metabolism and allergy

A person suffering from hepatolenticular degeneration or Wilson's disease stores excess copper in the liver, kidneys, brain, and cornea, leading to progressive destruction of the storing organ. Copper-containing IUDs should not be inserted in patients with this condition, or in any woman with an allergy to copper.

COMPLICATIONS

Syncope

Syncopal episodes have been associated with IUD insertion, especially in patients with a history of vasovagal problems. This may manifest as fainting, cardiac arrhythmias, seizures, or cardiac arrest. As the cause of such attacks is response to dilatation of the internal os, local anesthesia may prevent the occurrence. Prophylactic atropine has been used to prevent these attacks. Should such an attack occur after insertion, the patient should be placed in a horizontal position, the legs slightly elevated, vital functions supported, and if there is no rapid improvement, atropine should be administered and the IUD removed.

Expulsion

Expulsion of an IUD is most likely to occur during the first 3 months of use, especially during the first post-insertion menses. While the expulsion is often asymptomatic, there may be an episode of severe cramping and/or bleeding leading to expulsion. The IUD is more likely to be expelled if it fits poorly, i.e. one which is too large and is irritating to the uterus, leading to contractions and expulsion. The rate of expulsion decreases with advancing age, and with parity. There is a higher rate of expulsion with postpartum IUD insertion than if the IUD is inserted 3 months later, but in an unreliable patient population the IUD should be inserted as soon as possible. Every IUD wearer should be instructed to locate the IUD string before coitus at the end of each menses. She should be counseled that she is unprotected should the IUD be expelled, and that if her IUD string cannot be felt, she should use a barrier method until she can be examined.

Perforation

Transmyometrial perforations occur almost exclusively at the time of insertion. Transcervical perforations occur later, via uterine contractions. Diagnosis is made by careful search after the IUD string is lost. The endocervix is checked with a swab. If there is no possibility of pregnancy, an attempt may be made to find the IUD in the endometrial cavity with a hook or an alligator clamp. If no IUD is found, an ultrasound should be obtained. If ultrasound is unavailable, another IUD or a sound should be placed in the uterus and posterior–anterior and lateral X-rays obtained.

The diagnosis of perforation having been made, it must be decided whether to remove the IUD and by what means. Copper-containing IUDs may cause intense inflammation, adhesions, and scarring and must be removed. Progesterone-containing IUDs are suspected of causing similar problems and, therefore, should be removed. Inert closed IUDs such as the ring or bow must be removed due to the danger of bowel strangulation. Certain inert open IUDs (e.g. the Lippes loop) have been left in the peritoneal cavity without complication, but there are those who would argue that all IUDs must be removed (Lippes, 1978; Soderstrom, 1978).

IUDs embedded in the myometrium have been removed with the aid of the hysteroscope. Intraperitoneal IUDs may be removed using a laparoscope or culdoscope. If these means are unsuccessful, laparotomy must be performed.

Intrauterine pregnancy

The patient with an intrauterine pregnancy with an IUD in place should be advised to have the IUD removed. There is a 25% spontaneous abortion rate when this is done (Jennings, 1974; Lewit, 1970; Shine and Thompson, 1974; Tatum *et al.*, 1976). If the IUD is left in place, however, there is a 50% chance of spontaneous abortion, with an increased incidence of sepsis. This includes a peculiar type of septic midtrimester abortion associated with mortality (Cates *et al.*, 1976; Jennings, 1974). If the IUD string is not located, the uterus should not be probed. Rather, the pregnancy should be terminated if abortion is acceptable to the patient.

There are no known fetal anomalies with IUD use.

Ectopic pregnancy

Ectopic pregnancy may pose a greater danger to the woman wearing an IUD than to another individual, as her symptoms of pain and abnormal bleeding may be attributed to the IUD, and her real problem may be overlooked.

There is a higher ratio of ectopic to intrauterine pregnancies in IUD users than in the general population. This may be due only to the selective prevention of intrauterine pregnancies by the IUD and may not be a true increase in the incidence of ectopics. However, the increased incidence of inflammation of the fallopian tubes and alteration of tubal physiology may be responsible for a real increase in the incidence of tubal pregnancy.

Dysmenorrhea

There is an increase in two types of menstrual pain with IUD use; cramp-like pain as the uterus attempts to expel the IUD, and low backache.

Increased bleeding

The heaviest bleeding is reported in the first three cycles of IUD use. In subsequent cycles, there may be an acceptance by the patient of her increased flow. There is an increase in intermenstrual bleeding with IUD use, especially with the Progestasert. The intermenstrual bleeding is most likely to occur in the first few cycle days. An increase in menstrual bleeding occurs both in duration and in volume. The heaviest flow is reported with the inert IUDs (doubling of flow), with less increase with a copper-containing device (50% increase), while bleeding may even decrease with the Progestasert.

Pelvic inflammatory disease

PID may manifest as asymptomatic gonorrhea, endometritis, salpingitis, and salpingo-oophoritis with or without abscess formation. The incidence of all of these is increased with IUD use. Non-gonococcal PID, including actinomycosis, is increased to a greater degree (Eschenbach *et al.*, 1977; Faulkner and Ory, 1976; Henderson, 1973; Ledger, 1974; Ory, 1978; Schoen and Nowak, 1975; Targum and Wright, 1974).

The risk of infection occurs both at the time of IUD insertion and for the entire time the IUD is in place. Early diagnosis of PID in IUD wearers is sometimes missed. The symptoms may be attributed to the usual IUD side-effects.

When pelvic infection occurs in an IUD wearer who wishes for a subsequent pregnancy, she should be treated vigorously with antibiotics, the IUD removed, and another form of contraception chosen. If the patient wishes to have no further children, the IUD may be left in place unless it is a recurrent infection, or unless she has not responded to 48 hours of antibiotic therapy. In these circumstances, the IUD should be permanently removed. The long-term consequences of PID (infertility, ectopic pregnancy, adhesions, and chronic pelvic pain) must be considered.

Infertility

The patient who wishes to use an IUD and also wishes for further child-bearing should be warned, particularly if she is nulliparous, that her fertility may be compromised. This may occur secondary to PID, to tubal obstruction or to peritubal adhesions.

INSERTION

Candidacy

A woman wishing to use this method of contraception who has not been excluded by the above contraindications and who understands and accepts its possible complications is a candidate for IUD insertion.

Timing

During menstrual flow has been a generally accepted time of IUD insertion. The physician is reasonably confident that the patient is not pregnant. The cervical canal is slightly dilated at this time. The woman is already bleeding and thus is less likely to be alarmed by bleeding caused by insertion.

Some women may travel a great distance or have a great deal of inconvenience arranging child care or time away from work to consult a physician for IUD insertion. If the patient has been using a reliable method of contraception or has not had intercourse since her last menses, an IUD may be inserted any time in the cycle. The infection and expulsion rates may be less in such cases.

IUDs have been used postcoitally to prevent implantation. This is still considered an experimental procedure (ACOG Technical Bulletin, 1976; Lippes *et al.*, 1976).

Postpartum IUD insertion, shortly before hospital discharge, has a higher expulsion rate than does insertion later but initiates contraception, avoiding the possibility of pregnancy before the first postpartum office visit. If the IUD is expelled, a second IUD has a greater chance of being retained. New IUDs with chromic catgut suture projections are currently being tested for postpartum insertion. These show increased retention rates (Laufe *et al.*, 1979).

IUDs may be inserted immediately after abortion if the gestation was less than 12 weeks. Extra care must be taken to avoid perforation of the soft uterus.

Choice of IUD

The single most important factor in the choice of IUD is the competence and experience of the individual who undertakes the insertion. Fewer perforations, expulsions, and difficulties in insertion will be encountered if the practitioner is thoroughly familiar with the particular IUD.

The patient's ability to return for follow-up also influences the choice. Inert IUDs, such as the Lippes Loop or Saf-T-Coil, provide protection indefinitely. The copper-containing IUDs must be changed every 3 years. The Progestasert must be replaced yearly. In addition to the inconvenience and pain of frequent IUD changes, cost must be considered. The bioactive or medicated IUDs are usually more expensive.

The patient with a history of dysmenorrhea or menorrhagia is likely to tolerate a Progestasert best, with a copper-containing IUD the second best choice.

The obstetric history of the patient may influence the selection of IUD. A woman who has had a term vaginal delivery will probably accommodate any IUD. The woman who has had a caesarean section should have an IUD which is placed by withdrawal technique, rather than expulsion technique, i.e. a Saf-T-Coil or Cu-7 rather than a Lippes Loop. In a nulliparous woman who has had an early abortion and wishes to use an IUD, a small or medium Saf-T-Coil or a Lippes Loop A or B might be used. Nulligravid patients need IUDs with a small inserter barrel. The Cu-7 (3.07 mm) and the small Saf-T-Coil (3.76 mm) are smallest. Paracervical block should be considered for these women.

If the patient has a history of IUD expulsion, the uterine size should be reassessed. A more rigid IUD or a Progestasert may be considered superior.

The patient may request a particular IUD. If this occurs, she should be accommodated if possible. The patient will be much more compliant and have many fewer complaints if she is comfortable with the IUD chosen.

Explanation and instructions

Before IUD insertion the patient needs good counseling. Simple, easily understandable language should be used. The counselor should be a sympathetic, well-informed individual who is candid about possible complications, but not alarming. This should not be a hurried session, and the patient should be encouraged to ask questions. Other contraceptive methods should be explained and offered.

A description of the insertion process must be included. The patient should be told that she may experience some pain, cramping, nausea, bleeding, or fainting. She should be encouraged to have someone accompany her on the day of insertion.

The patient must know of the possible complications of IUD use. She should know that the IUD may fail to prevent pregnancy, and what will be recommended should this happen. She should be warned of increased menstrual complaints, including increased flow, cramping, long menses, spotting, and anemia. She must be made aware of the possibility of infection and its consequences, i.e. increased incidence of ectopic pregnancy, infertility, and (if untreated) abscesses and possible need for hysterectomy. She needs to know the risk of perforation and how she will be medically managed should this occur.

Responsibility for the health of the patient is shared by the health-care provider and the patient. She must be told of her duties after an IUD is inserted. If her IUD is lost, she will not know it is happening. She must check monthly for her IUD string. If it is not felt, she must use a barrier method of contraception until she is examined. If the IUD itself is felt, she should proceed as if the IUD has been lost. She should never pull on the IUD string or let anyone else pull on it. She should call immediately if she experiences unexplained fever, pelvic pain or tenderness, severe cramping, unusual bleeding, heavy discharge, problems in checking the string, or if menses are missed. The follow-up care which is planned should be thoroughly understood. The next appointment should be made before the patient leaves the office. When the IUD needs to be changed, which IUD is being used and the telephone number to call should problems arise should be written on a card which the patient should carry with her. If the patient wishes to have the IUD removed it may be done at any time, but if she does not wish to become pregnant the IUD should not be removed midcycle after having had intercourse. All IUDs should be removed after the menopause. Every woman with an IUD needs an annual check-up which includes Pap smear, breast examination, and hematocrit.

Process of insertion

The following steps should be performed:

(1) Administer analgesic or sedative if necessary.
(2) Administer atropine if syncope is expected from a history of vasovagal symptoms.
(3) Perform speculum examination. Inspect. Do Pap smear and gonorrhea culture. Remove speculum.

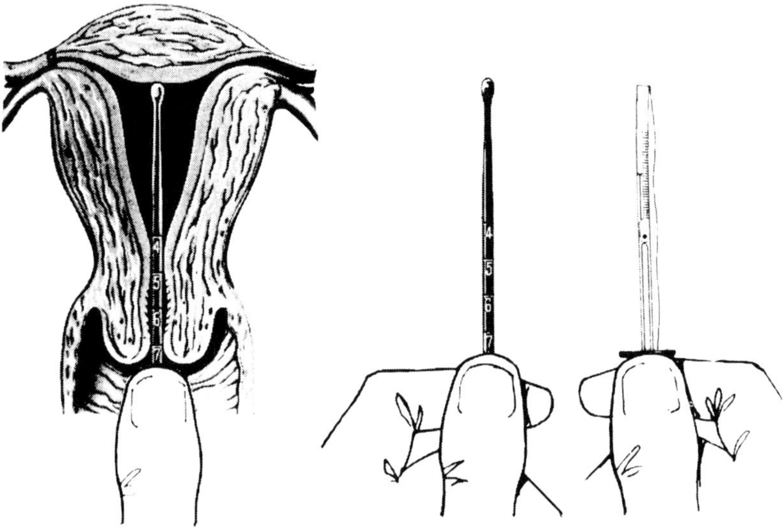

Figure 5.1 Sounding of the uterus to determine which IUD is best, and to what depth the IUD should be inserted

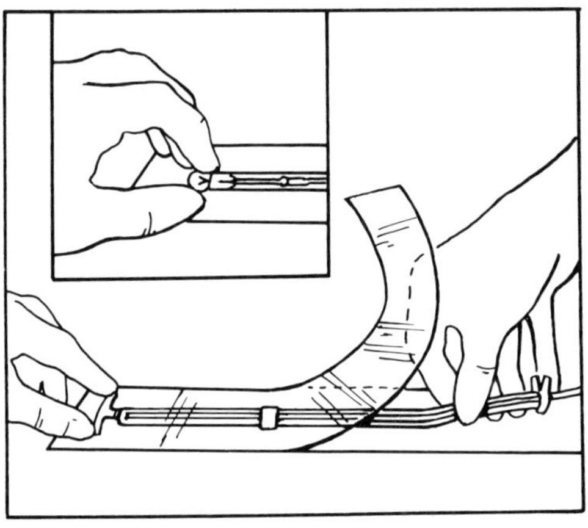

Figure 5.2 Loading of the IUD in sterile conditions

(4) Do bimanual examination. Examine uterus for size, shape, position, and mobility. Examine adnexa for masses or tenderness, to rule out malignancy or infection. Perform rectovaginal examination, again looking for masses or tenderness.

(5) Change gloves.

(6) Proceed with second sterile speculum examination. Wash the cervix with antiseptic. Cleanse the endocervix with a swab saturated with antiseptic.

(7) Administer anesthetic if necessary. This is likely to be the case with the nullipara or patient with known cervical stenosis. Check for lidocaine allergy first. Warn the patient of possible nausea, dizziness, and tingling lips. Swab the cervix with a swab saturated with lidocaine. Insert needle just under mucosa in connective tissue at the 4:00 position. Aspirate slightly. Inject 5 cm^3 lidocaine. Repeat at the 8:00 position. Wait 5 minutes for anesthesia to occur.

(8) Place tenaculum on the anterior lip of the cervix approximately 1.5 cm from the os. Use the tenaculum to straighten the uterus, correcting flexion and stabilizing the uterus.

(9) Sound the uterus to make the final decision on which is the proper IUD (Figure 5.1). If the uterus sounds less than 4.5 cm, no IUD will fit. If the uterus measures 4.5–6.5 cm, a vertical length less than 3 cm is needed, therefore a small Saf-T-Coil is proper. If a measurement of 6.5–9.9 cm is obtained, any IUD will do. If the uterus is over 10 cm, a large Saf-T-Coil or large Lippes Loop, Cu-7, or Progestasert may be used, but a second means of contraception should be recommended.

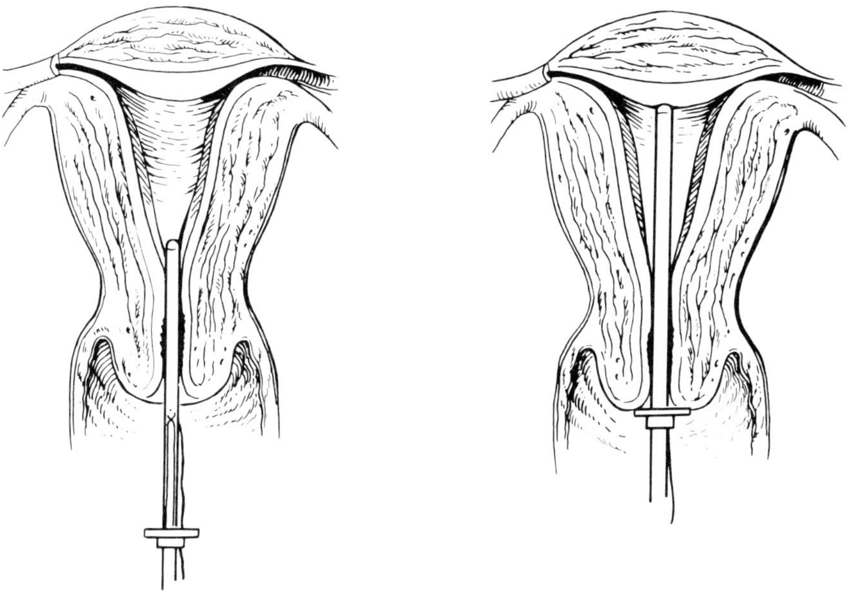

Figure 5.3 Insertion of the barrel high into the fundus

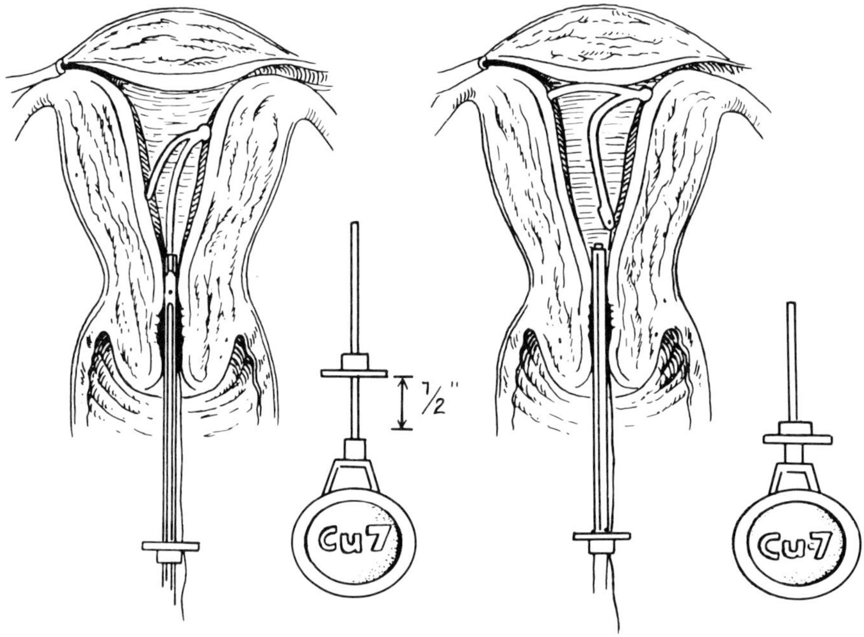

Figure 5.4 Insertion of an IUD with the push method

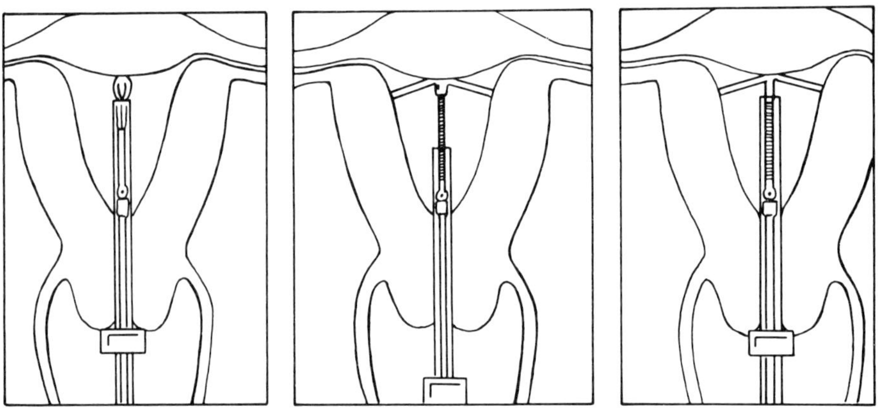

Figure 5.5 Insertion of an IUD with the withdrawal technique

(10) Load the IUD under sterile conditions (Figure 5.2). Proceed quickly, as the IUD will lose its resilience if it is in the inserter too long.

(11) Place traction on the tenaculum, straightening and stabilizing the uterus once again.

(12) Insert the barrel high into the fundus for the fewest pregnancies and the least chance of expulsion (Figure 5.3).
(13) *Slowly* insert the IUD. If an IUD is being inserted with the push method, push the plunger into the barrel, pushing the IUD out into the uterine cavity (Figure 5.4). If an IUD which allows insertion by the withdrawal technique is being used, retract the outer barrel over the plunger, leaving the IUD in place (Figure 5.5.).
(14) Withdraw the inserter apparatus.
(15) Clip the strings long. They can always be shortened later.
(16) Remove the speculum.
(17) Teach the patient how to find the IUD string. Make sure she has located it.
(18) Repeat that spotting and/or cramping are not unusual.
(19) Answer any questions the patient has.
(20) Allow her to lie quietly until all pain has subsided.
(21) See the patient in 6 weeks to 3 months, then at least yearly.

In conclusion, the IUD is an effective means of contraception if the patient is a good candidate, the IUD is properly chosen and inserted, and follow-up care and counseling are adequate.

References

ACOG Technical Bulletin (1976). *The Intrauterine Device.* No. 40

Cates, W., Ory, H. W., Rochat, R. W. and Tyler, C. W. (1976). The intrauterine device and deaths from spontaneous abortion. *N. Engl. J. Med.,* **295**, 1155

Eschenbach, D. A., Harnisch, J. P. and Holmes, K. K. (1977). Pathogenesis of acute pelvic inflammatory disease: role of contraception and other risk factors. *Am. J. Obstet. Gynecol.,* **128**, 838

Faulkner, W. L. and Ory, H. W. (1976). Intrauterine devices and acute pelvic inflammatory disease. *J. Am. Med. Assoc.,* **235**, 1851

Henderson, S. R. (1973). Pelvic actinomycosis associated with an intrauterine device. *Obstet. Gynecol.,* **41**, 726

Jennings, J. (1974). *Report of Safety and Efficacy of the Dalkon Shield and Other IUDs,* p. 19. (New York: FDA Ad Hoc Obstetric-Gynecology Advisory Committee

Laufe, L. E., Wheeler, R. G. and Friel, P. G. (1979). Modification of intrauterine devices for postpartum insertion. *Lancet,* **1**, 853

Ledger, W. J. (1974). Relationship of pelvic infection to various types of contraception. *Clin. Obstet. Gynecol.,* **17**, 79

Lewit, S. (1970). Outcome of pregnancy with intrauterine devices. *Contraception,* **2**, 47

Lippes, J. (1978). Management of the lost IUD: a conservative approach. In Sciarra, J. J., Zatuchni, G. E. and Speidel, J. J. (eds.) *Risks, Benefits and Controversies in Fertility Control,* p. 404. (Hagerstown, Md.: Harper and Row)

Lippes, J., Malik, T. and Tatum, H. J. (1976). The postcoital copper-T. *Adv. Planned Parenthood,* **11**, 24

Luukkainen, T. and Nilsson, C. G. (1978). Sustained intrauterine release of d-Norgestrel. *Contraception,* **18**, 451

Ory, H. W. (1978). A review of the association between intrauterine devices and acute pelvic inflammatory disease. *J. Reprod. Med.,* **20**, 200

Rybo, G. and Bergqvist, A. (1978). Comparison of menstrual blood loss with the Progestasert system and the Cu-T-200; preliminary results. In Mishell, D. R., Jr. and Martinez, J. (eds.) *Proceedings of a Symposium on Clinical Experience with the Progesterone Uterine Therapeutic System,* p. 106. (Princeton, N.J.: Excerpta Medica)

Schoen, J. A. and Nowak, R. J. (1975). Repeat ectopic pregnancy, A 16-year clinical survey. *Obstet. Gynecol.,* **45**, 542

Shine, R. M. and Thompson, J. F. (1974). The *in situ* IUD and pregnancy outcome. *Am. J. Obstet. Gynecol.,* **119**, 124

Soderstrom, R. M. (1978). The wandering IUD: what to do. In Sciarra, J. J., Zatuchni, G. I. and Speidel, J. J. (eds.) *Risks, Benefits and Controversies in Fertility Control,* p. 480. (Hagerstown, Md.: Harper and Row)

Tatum, H. J., Schmidt, F. H. and Jain, A. K. (1976). Management and outcome of pregnancies associated with the Copper T intrauterine contraceptive device. *Am. J. Obstet. Gynecol.,* **126**, 869

Targum, S. D. and Wright, N. H. (1974). Association of the intrauterine device and pelvic inflammatory disease: a retrospective pilot study. *Am. J. Epidemiol.,* **100**, 262

Zador, S., Nilsson, B. A., Nilsson, B., Sjoberg, N. O., Westrom, L. and Wiese, J. (1976). Clinical experience with the uterine progesterone system (Progestasert). *Contraception,* **13**, 559

6
Interception by postcoital insertion of an IUD

M. R. VAN SANTEN AND A. A. HASPELS

INTRODUCTION

After the development of postcoital hormonal interception in the 1960s with diethylstilbestrol in the USA (Morris and Van Wagenen, 1966) and ethinyl estradiol in Europe (Haspels, 1969), Tatum in the early 1970s proposed a postcoital method of interception with IUDs that successfully prevents pregnancy and then continues to provide contraceptive protection. The major advantage of this treatment is that it avoids the use of a massive dose of estrogens, a very effective postcoital method, but associated with nausea and vomiting. The method is used up to 5 days after exposure; this is an extension of 3 days in comparison with the estrogen treatment, and provides continuing contraception in women who leave the IUD in place.

A major disadvantage of postcoital IUD use is that if a patient has a gonococcal infection or pelvic inflammatory disease (PID), IUD insertion can produce serious complications. This depends largely on the behavior of the patient and the local VD rate of the community. Cases of rape are excluded from these services for this reason, but if they present early a proper check-up and treatment can be done within the 5 days available for this method and a postcoital IUD can still be inserted. The potential risk of future fertility is to be considered as the incidence of PID in nulliparous IUD users is seven times higher compared with multiparous women and nine times greater compared with non-users. Women below 25 years of age are found to be more prone to infections, and approximately 70% of women asking for interception are nulliparous and younger than 25 years. Another important disadvantage is the risk of septic abortion if the IUD is inserted in a woman who has become pregnant. Septic abortion is a life-threatening condition.

The continuation rate is 78% among young nulliparous women because of discomfort and side-effects. The disadvantages that exist with IUDs in general must be considered. These include vasovagal reflexes with nausea, vomiting, bradycardia, or syncope at the time of insertion. Out of several series no pregnancies are reported in the month of treatment. The preferred IUD is the Multiload Copper IUD or the Copper T; the high expulsion rate proves the Copper 7 inefficient.

In suitable circumstances, the IUD is the first choice of postcoital interception.

POSTCOITAL ESTROGENS

Up to today hormonal postcoital contraception is prescribed by using estrogens, in Europe ethinyl estradiol 5 mg/day (Haspels, 1976) and in the USA mostly diethylstilbestrol (DES) 50 mg per day for 5 consecutive days is used (Morris and Van Wagenen, 1966).

IUD

Using IUDs for family-planning management has become a general practice, yet as a postcoital interceptive technique it is not yet commonly in use. Insertion of an IUD so as to interfere with a possible pregnancy as a consequence of a non-protected coital act was first proposed in the early 1970s by Tatum (Lippes *et al.*, 1976).

MECHANISM OF ACTION

Spermatozoa proceed quickly through the uterus to the fallopian tubes after sexual intercourse. Within 15 minutes after deposit of semen in the posterior vaginal pouch, spermatozoa reach the fimbrial part of the fallopian tube (Settlage *et al.*, 1973). No interceptive action is expected from the sperm-destroying effect of an IUD. Neither ovulation nor capacitation is prevented.

Endocrine mechanisms interfering with pregnancy induced by the IUD have been searched for. Cytologic smears from the vagina show a low pycnotic index, suggesting a short luteal phase in IUD users. Luteolysis is supposed to be possible by the action of prostaglandin $PGF_{2\alpha}$, liberated by laceration of the endometrial surface. Enhanced tubal motility through the prostaglandin intermediate causes the oocyte to arrive too early in the uterine cavity, in asynchrony with the endometrium (Czernobilsky *et al.*, 1975). This causes the ovum to perish (Chang, 1950). The effectiveness of postcoital estrogens is thought to be due to a similar mechanism (Van Santen and Haspels, 1980; Morris and Van Wagenen, 1973). IUDs in mice induce a proliferative stage of the endometrium. Copper in rabbit and cats induces proliferative-like stroma in the endometrium by which asynchrony by endometrium delay is achieved.

The insertion of an IUD contaminates the uterine cavity for at least 24 hours, but usually for several days (Huber *et al.*, 1980). A blastocidal effect through bacterial infection or the reactions to it seems likely in the postcoital use of an IUD; however, in continuing contraception by IUD, inflammatory reactions are not a mechanism of action (Zipper *et al.*, 1977).

The copper dispersion in the first month of use is important for the postcoital use. In mouse an *in vitro* concentration of 2.5×10^{-5} mol/l is thought to be embryotoxic (Brinster and Cross, 1972). IUDs with a 200 mm^2 copper surface area yield, by release of copper ions, a concentration of 9×10^{-4} mol/l in the uterine cavity (Oster, 1971). Copper release is high during the first months after insertion. The high efficacy of the postcoital IUCuD might be explained by the high embryotoxic copper ion concentration in the uterine cavity in contrast with the inert IUD with its maximum pregnancy rates in the first months of use (Tietze and Lewit, 1970). *In vitro* studies show inhibition of fetal growth by copper, and no influence is seen with inert IUDs (Jones *et al.*, 1973).

CONTRACEPTIVE EFFICACY

The postcoital use of an IUD has proved to be very effective. In a series of 326 women (Lippes *et al.*, 1976, 1979), no pregnancies have been reported. In India 1039 interval insertions have been reported at family planning stations, and in a series of 250 patients with a follow-up of 96.2% a pregnancy rate of 0.9% was found, but insertion was done just at the day of visit to the clinic irrespective of the date of the menstrual cycle or of coitus. Recently a British study of 200 women reported 100% efficacy. First studies mention the use of the Cu-7 Gravigard IUD, especially in the nulliparous patient (Eliot and McGregor, 1978). Later the Cu-T-200 was suggested (Lippes *et al.*, 1976), but an expulsion rate after 1 month of use in the nulliparous of 1.7 was found, and a discontinuation rate of 10.7 (Mishell *et al.*, 1973). The pregnancy rate of the Cu-7 Gravigard IUD was found to be 2.8 (Gini, 1978). In the nulliparous the expulsion rate is most in the first 3 months of use (Newton *et al.*, 1974). This phenomenon led to the use of other types of IUD. The lowest expulsion rate so far was found with the Multiload Cu250 IUD (Van Os *et al.*, 1978; Sadovsky and Yarkoni, 1978). No relationship between the day of the menstrual cycle on which insertion of Cu-T-200 or Cu-7 Gravigard IUDs took place and continuation or termination rates could be demonstrated (White *et al.*, 1980; Edelman *et al.*, 1979). Initially, no difference was found in pregnancy rate according to time of insertion in the menstrual cycle (Akinla *et al.*, 1975) but in recent studies of over 9000 interval insertions the pregnancy rate was found to be halved if insertion took place after day 11 of the menstrual cycle, in comparison with insertion during the bleeding phase of menstruation (White *et al.*, 1980).

ADVANTAGES OF POSTCOITAL IUD INSERTION

Several investigators have used the postcoital copper IUD as the method of choice in postcoital interception practice (*Drug and Therapeutics Bulletin*, 1980), provided circumstances favored such a procedure and the women had a stable relationship. The main advantage is the continuing contraception achieved by the IUD. A continuation rate of 78% was found in one such series (Yuzpe, 1979); and an IUCuD can be left in place as long as 5 years, without being less effective (Huber *et al.*, 1980).

With the declining efficacy of postcoital estrogens after 36 hours postcoitum, the postcoital technique of insertion of an IUD provides interception up to 5 days, since in women the ovum transport to the uterine cavity takes 4–5 days (Croxatto *et al.*, 1972). Intrauterine techniques of removal of the embryo, with the risk of endometrial damage, are avoided. This technique is slightly uncomfortable for some patients but for all no high dosage of estrogens needs to be taken. Even with such a 5-day course of estrogens, no protection against pregnancy is provided after further intercourse. In all cases in which estrogens are contraindicated – such as patients with a history of previous thrombosis, hepatic disease, and mammary or ovarian neoplasms – the postcoital IUD insertion supplies a good, non-hormonal alternative to prevent pregnancy.

DISADVANTAGES OF POSTCOITAL IUD INSERTION

In comparison with the regular use of an IUD, the postcoital technique of insertion is much more complicated. First of all, the midcycle insertion differs from the usual late-menstrual, since the cervical canal is tender, and less wide. The periovulatory internal ostium can be passed easily, but pre- and postovulatory it is sometimes tight and rigid (especially in nulliparas), so insertion becomes painful and hazardous. An occasional cardiac arrest associated with insertion of an IUD is described, while the syncope resulting from vagal reflexes is known to all physicians practicing IUD insertions (Aznar *et al.*, 1976).

Lessening of pain and possibly averting bradycardia and hypotension is easily achieved by paracervical injection of a local anesthetic, and administration of atropine is optional if patients have a history of fainting easily. This technique is described in detail by Lippes *et al.* (1976). In our series, local anesthetics were used only occasionally in nulliparous patients, since multiparous women always allowed an easy postcoital insertion without discomfort.

Secondly, the need for an IUD is unexpected to the patient, and she will feel embarrassed (Huggins *et al.*, 1979). This has to be taken into account, and the doctor does not have the opportunity to prepare the patient for such an insertion. The patient's history must be taken carefully and the risk of venereal infection must be judged mostly on the circumstances only. Doubt about the partner makes the proposed technique unsuitable, because of fear of infections. So in cases of rape postcoital insertion of an IUD is not recommended, but estrogens should be given – the management known as 'morning-after pill' and described earlier. If the patient reports for treatment early after the accident she is treated adequately first, if needed, and she receives the IUD later. The menstrual history must exclude any possibility of an early pregnancy. A pregnancy test or ultrasound scanning must be considered in case of any doubt. Life-threatening septic abortions due to an IUD *in situ* are well known (Cates *et al.*, 1976). IUD insertion when menstruation is delayed (*British Medical Journal*, 1976) must be rejected for this reason. Endometrial aspiration before day 25 of the menstrual cycle, or within 10 days of unprotected intercourse (Eliot and McGregor, 1978), or an early menstrual extraction must be considered instead. Postcoital IUD insertion will often be requested by nulliparous women. No reduced fertility is found after IUD use as such, provided no complications occur (Tietze, 1968). There has been no consensus about IUD use and ectopic pregnancy risks, but recent published results show this to be unlikely (Haspels and Thiery, 1980).

As no pregnancies with postcoital use of IUD have been reported, the matter of ectopic pregnancies with this method remains undiscussed.

PELVIC INFLAMMATORY DISEASE

Multiple sexual partners are considered an additional risk factor for PID (Flesh *et al.*, 1979). This must be considered when taking the history of the patient. Besides gonorrhea, more or less abundant vaginal discharge or even cervicitis might be found on examination. Non-gonococcal infections are, even when properly treated, potential hazards. More tubal occlusions occur through non-gonococcal salpingitis. An infection occurring for the first time causes closed tubes in 13% of cases, with a recurrence rate of 20%; a second PID results in 35.5% infertility owing to tubal obstruction. PID occurs seven times more often in nulliparous IUD users than in non-users (Weström *et al.*, 1976). The risk of infection is increased with insertion in the latter half of the secretory phase of the menstrual cycle, e.g. after the 22nd day (Akinla *et al.*, 1975). No index is found for a high infection risk at midcycle. Contrastingly, hysterosalpingography performed midcycle hardly ever results in infections, provided a proper aseptic technique is used.

OTHER FACTORS

A hazard to be kept in mind is rheumatic heart disease. Bacterial endocarditis may not be mentioned by the doctor while taking the history, nor mentioned by the patient in the stress of asking for postcoital interception (Huggins *et al.*, 1979). This can result in lethal complications, as insertion of an IUD apparently causes bacteremia (De Swiet *et al.*, 1975).

In modern gynecologic practice, it is routine to collect cytologic specimens from the cervix before inserting an IUD. In case of postcoital need for interception the time lapse available can be used for laboratory tests and evaluation of cytologic and, if needed, bacteriologic samples.

From studies in rats, it is found the IUD needs to be present only on the days of nidation (Segal, 1971). Insertion with removal *before* nidation and insertion with removal *after* nidation, has no direct contraceptive effect on the oocyte (Joshi and Gunn, 1971). Clinicians are aware that removal of an IUD in the secretory phase of the menstrual cycle has a chance to allow a uterine pregnancy to develop which otherwise would have been prevented (Strickler, 1978).

In our series of postcoital IUD insertions, we selected only women who have had intercourse with their regular partner. Insertion was performed only if vaginal discharge and palpatory findings of the internal sexual organs were normal. All insertions took place within 5 days of unprotected intercourse. Initially, Cu-7 Gravigard IUD and Cu-T-200 IUD were used, because of their convenient insertion technique. After treatment of nine patients with a Cu-T-200 or Cu-7 Gravigard IUD only insertion with Multi-

Table 6.1 Number (%) of IUDs inserted postcoitally[a]

No. (%) of patients	*Type of IUD used*			
	ML Cu 375	*ML Cu 250*	*Cu 7*	*Cu T*
50 (100)	34 (68)	7 (14)	6(12)	3(6)

[a] There were no pregnancies, apart from one patient who conceived in the second month after IUD insertion.

load type IUD was performed. The division is shown in Table 6.1.

Though no pregnancies have occurred in the treatment month, we later found a partial expulsion of the Cu-7 Gravigard IUD in the month after insertion, unnoticed by the patient, and the patient had become pregnant in the meantime. Exact dating of the pregnancy was done by ultrasound scanning, which showed that the pregnancy did not date from a conception in the month of treatment. The Cu-7 Gravigard IUD has a high expulsion rate of approximately 10% (Bernstein *et al.*, 1972). A rate of 17%, including partial expulsion, has been noted (Haspels, unpublished observations). For this reason the use of Cu-7 Gravigard IUD was abandoned and the study continued with insertion of Multiload Cu-250 IUD only, since very low expulsion rates have been reported. We noticed that insertion of the Multiload IUD in the periovulatory period was very easy, despite the different structure of this IUD. Later on we were supplied with Multiload Cu-375 IUD, which we now use exclusively.

Table 6.2 shows the results of the postcoital tests performed on the latter 19 patients in our series and the parity of our patients.

Table 6.2 Parity and results of postcoital tests performed on last 19 patients in series. Percentages are given in parentheses

Cervical mucus test for spermatozoa		*Parity*		
Present	*Not present*	*0*	*1*	*2*
15 (79)	4(21)	12(63)	4(21)	3(16)

CONCLUDING REMARKS

The use of an IUD postcoitally has proved to be a good alternative to the massive dose of estrogens usually provided to the women seeking help in postcoital prevention of pregnancy.

The circumstances should favour such an insertion; risk of infection, or possibly existing pregnancy, will endanger the patient if an insertion is performed. The general health of the women is to be checked carefully, since endocarditis might worsen if not properly dealt with. Estrogen contraindication can be honored by the alternative of inserting a postcoital IUD.

The emotional stress of patients otherwise needing the morning-after pill might be augmented by this invasive technique but they are secure from the high dosage of estrogens, with strong side-effects, needed for high efficacy.

Contraception by postcoital IUD insertion is highly effective. In the documented series of postcoital insertions, no pregnancies have yet been reported, whereas in midcycle exposure, the chance of becoming pregnant is estimated as 20% (Tietze, 1960).

The postcoital IUD insertion procedure is a means of interception after the time for postcoital estrogen has elapsed. With this method endometrial aspiration or even therapeutic abortion may be avoided.

The continuing contraception achieved with the postcoital IUD provides protection against pregnancy after further intercourse. The lower termination rate after midcycle insertion supports the belief that the postcoital IUD is a superior means of interception in comparison with postcoital estrogen administration. Therefore, given favorable circumstances, postcoital IUD insertion is often the first choice of interception.

Acknowledgment

The use of Multiload Cu-375 IUDs in the patients of our study was made possible by donated supplies from Organon Nederland, Oss, The Netherlands.

References

Akinla, O., Luukkainen, T. and Timonen, H. (1975). Important factors in the use effectiveness of the Copper-T-200 IUD. *Contraception*, **12**, 697

Aznar, R., Reynoso, L., Ley, E., Gamez, R. and Diaz De Leon, M. (1976). Electrocardiographic changes induced by insertion of an intrauterine device and other uterine manipulations. *Fertil. Steril.*, **27**, 92

Bernstein, G. S., Israel, R., Seward, P. and Mishell, D. R., Jr. (1972). Clinical experience with the Cu-7 intrauterine device. *Contraception*, **6**, 99

Brinster, R. I. and Cross, P. C. (1972). Effect of copper on the preimplantation mouse embryo. *Nature*, **238**, 398

British Medical Journal. (1976). Postcoital contraception. *Br. Med. J.*, **1**, 961

Cates, W., Jr., Ory, H. W., Rochat, R. W. and Tyler, C. W. (1976). The intrauterine device and deaths from spontaneous abortion. *N. Engl. J. Med.*, **295**, 1115

Chang, M. C. (1950). Development and fate of transferred rabbit ova or blastocyst in relation to the ovulation time of recipients. *J. Exp. Zool.*, **114**, 197

Croxatto, H. B., Diaz, S., Fuentealba, B., Croxatto, H. D., Carrillo, D. and Fabres, C. (1972). Studies on the duration of egg transport in the human oviduct. Part I. The time between ovulation and egg recovery from the uterus in normal women. *Fertil. Steril.*, **23**, 447

Czernobilsky, B., Rotenstreich, L., Mass, N. and Lancet, M. (1975). Effect of intrauterine device on histology of endometrium. *Obstet. Gynecol.*, **45**, 64

De Swiet, M., Ramsay, I. D. and Rees, G. M. (1975). Bacterial endocarditis after insertion of intrauterine contraceptive device. *Br. Med. J.*, **3**, 76

Drug and Therapeutics Bulletin (1980). Postcoital contraception. *Drug Ther. Bull.*, **18**, 5

Edelman, D. A., Zipper, J., Rivera, M. and Medel, M. (1979). Timing of the IUD insertion. *Contraception*, **19**, 449

Eliot, J. W. and McGregor, D. (1978). Postcoital contraception by endometrial aspiration. *Adv. Planned Parenthood*, **13**, 21

Flesh, G., Weiner, J. M., Corlett, R. C., Jr., Boice, C., Mishell, D. R., Jr. and Wolf, R. M. (1979). The intrauterine contraceptive device and acute salpingitis. A multifactor analysis. *Am. J. Obstet. Gynecol.*, **135**, 402

Gini, P. C. (1978). An analysis of the use of Copper-7 intrauterine contraceptive device. *Nigerian Med. J.*, **8**, 319

Haspels, A. A. (1969) 9th abstract, 6th world congress on obstetics and gynecology, New York. *Int. J. Gynecol. Obstet.*, **8**, 113

Haspels, A. A. (1976). Interception: postcoital estrogens in 3016 women. *Contraception*, **14**, 375

Haspels, A. A. and Thiery, M. (1980). IUDs and extrauterine pregnancy. In Hafez, E. and van Os, W. A. A. (eds.) *IUD Pathology and Management*. Progress in Contraceptive Delivery Systems vol. III, p. 187 (Lancaster: MTP Press)

Huber, A., Mikuz, G. and Colleselli, K. (1980). Langzeitbeobachtungen zur wirkung von Kupfer-Intrauterin-Pessaren. *Geburtsh. u. Frauenheilk.*, **39**, 857

Huggins, G. R., Rosenfeld, D. L., Rickels, K., Garcia, C.-R. and Fisher, E. L. (1979). Emotional distress in morning-after pill patients. *Acta Obstet. Gynecol. Scand.*, **58**, 65

Jones, R. W., Gregson, N. M. and Einstein, M. (1973). Effect of copper-containing intrauterine devices on human cells in culture. *Br. Med. J.*, **2**, 520

Joshi, S. G., and Gunn, B. A. (1971). Effects of postcoital insertion of an intrauterine foreign body in rats. *Contraception*, **3**, 401

Lippes, J., Malik, T. and Tatum, H. J. (1976). The post coital copper T. *Adv. Planned Parenthood*, **11**, 24

Lippes, J., Tatum, H. J., Maulid, D. and Zielezny, M. (1979). Postcoital copper IUD found to be effective in preventing pregnancy. *Fam. Planning Perspectives*, **11**, 195

Mishell, D. R., Israel, R. and Freid, N. (1973). A study of the copper-T intrauterine contraceptive device TCu200 in nulliparous women. *Am. J. Obstet. Gynecol.*, **116**, 1092

Morris, J. McL. and Van Wagenen, G. (1966). Compounds interfering with ovum implantation and development. III The role of estrogens. *Am. J. Obstet. Gynecol.*, **96**, 804

Morris, J. McL. and Van Wagenen, G. (1973). Interception: the use of postovulatory estrogens, to prevent implantation. *Am. J. Obstet. Gynecol.*, **115**, 101

Newton, J., Elias, J., McEwan, J. and Mann, G. (1974). Intrauterine contraception with the copper seven: evaluation after two years. *Br. Med. J.*, **3**, 447

Oster, G. K. (1971). Reaction of metallic copper with biological substrates. *Nature*, **234**, 153

Sadovsky, E. and Yarkoni, S. (1978). Preliminary report on the use of the combined Multiload Contraceptive intrauterine device (MLCu-250). *Fertil. Steril.*, **30**, 529

Segal, S. J. (1971). Intrauterine devices and their mechanism of action. In Diczfalusy, E. and Borell, U. (eds.) *Control of Human Fertility* (Proceedings of the 15th Nobel Symposium, Sweden), p. 181. (Stockholm: Almqvist & Wiksell)

Settlage, D. S. F., Motoshima, M. and Tredway, D. R. (1973). Sperm transport from the external cervical os to the fallopian tubes in women: a time and quantitation study. *Fertil. Steril.*, **24**, 655

Strickler, R. C. (1978). Elective removal of an intrauterine device. *Can. Med. Assoc. J.*, **118**, 1028

Tietze, C. (1960). Probability of pregnancy resulting from a single unprotected coitus. *Fertil. Steril.*, **11**, 485

Tietze, C. (1968). Fertility after discontinuation of intrauterine and oral contraception. *Int. J. Fertil.*, **13**, 385

Tietze, C. and Lewis, S. (1970). Evaluation of intrauterine devices: Ninth Progress Report of the Cooperative Statistical Program. *Stud. Fam. Plann.*, **55**, 1

van Os, W. A. A., De Nooyer, C. C. A., Bakker, S., Bomert, L., Rhemrev, P. E. R. and Loendersloot, E. W. (1978). Evaluation of the combined Multiload Copper IUD (ML Cu 250 and ML Cu 375). *Int. J. Fertil.*, **23**, 152

Van Santen, M. R. and Haspels, A. A. (1980). Interfering with implantation by postcoital estrogen administration. I. Endometrium Histology. In Leroy, F., Finn, C. A., Psychoyos, A. and Hubinont, P. O. (eds.) *Progress in Reproductive Biology*, p. 310 (Basel Karger)

Weström, I., Bengtsson, L. P. and Mardh, P. (1976). The risk of pelvic inflammatory disease in women using intrauterine contraceptive devices as compared to non-users. *Lancet*, **2**, 221

White, M. K., Ory, H. W., Rooks, J. B. and Rochat, R. W. (1980). Intrauterine device termination rates and the menstrual cycle day of insertion. *Obstet. Gynecol.*, **55**, 220

Yuzpe, A. A. (1979). Postcoital contraception. *Int. J. Gynaecol. Obstet.*, **16**, 497

Zipper, J., Edelman, D. A. and Goldsmith, A. (1977). An overview of IUD research and implications for the future. *Int. J. Gynaecol. Obstet.*, **15**, 73

7
Diagnosis and management of IUD with missing tail

A. H. ANSARI AND V. M. ANSARI

Uterine perforation resulting in displacement of an IUD within the abdominal cavity occurs with an incidence of 0.2–8.7 per 1000 insertions

Table 7.1 **Etiology, diagnosis, and management of IUD with missing tail**

ETIOLOGY

(1) Retraction within the uterine cavity:
- Short tail
- Device rotation
- Polar change

(2) Elective removal of tail to avoid expulsion

(3) Unnoticed expulsion

(4) Uterine growth:
- Pregnancy
- Tumor

(5) Uterine perforation:
- Incomplete extrusion
- Complete extrusion

DIAGNOSIS

(1) Uterine exploration:
- Cervical canal
- Uterine cavity

(2) Flat plate of the abdomen

(3) Hysterosalpingogram

(4) Pelvic pneumogram

(5) Ultrasonography

MANAGEMENT

Occult		*Displaced*	
(1)	Polyp forceps	(1)	Laparotomy
(2)	Uterine hook	(2)	Laporoscopy
(3)	Serrated tip curette	(3)	Culdoscopy
(4)	Dilatation and curettage	(4)	Culdotomy
(5)	Hysteroscopy		
(6)	MI-Mark		

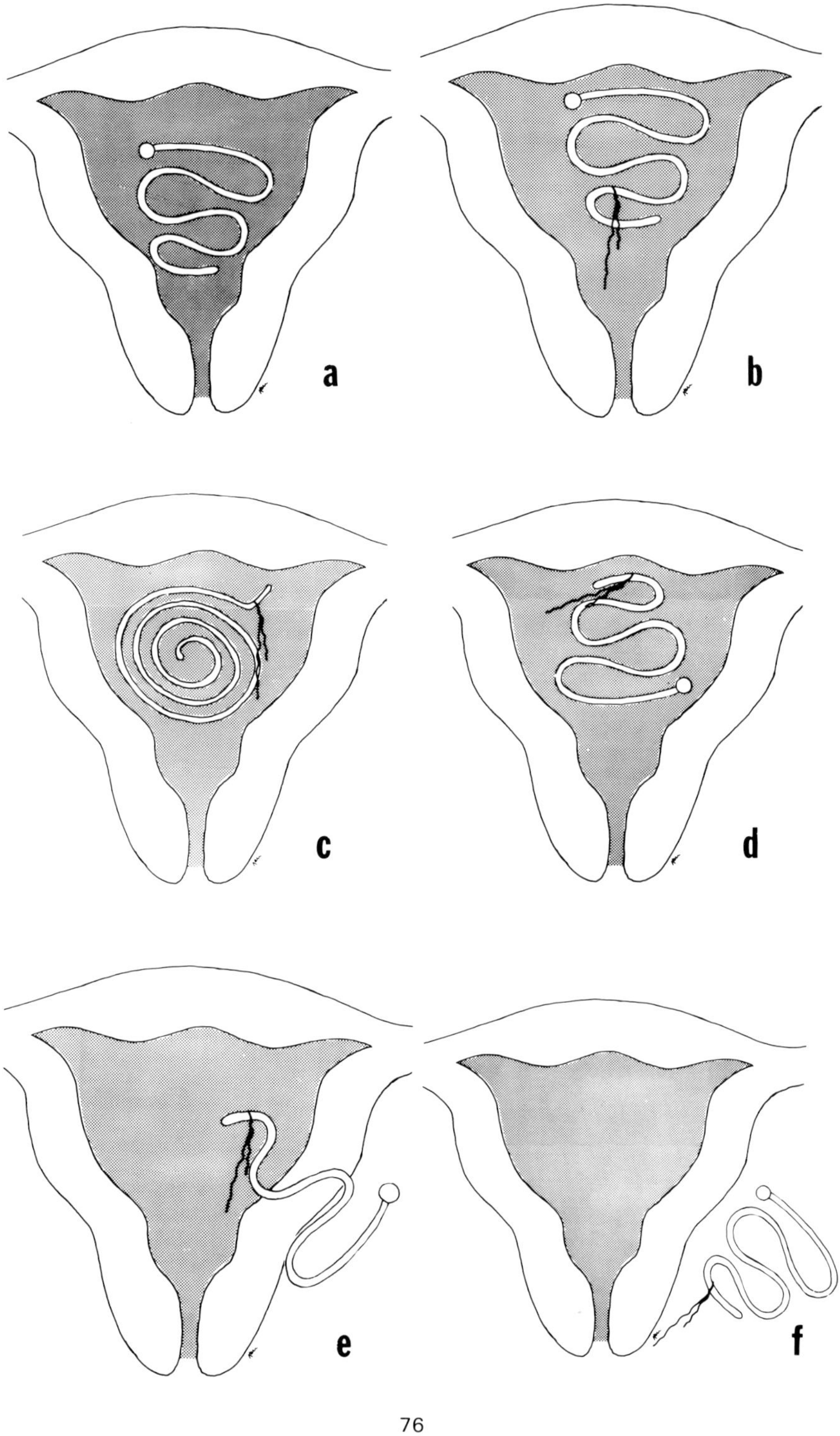
a
b
c
d
e
f

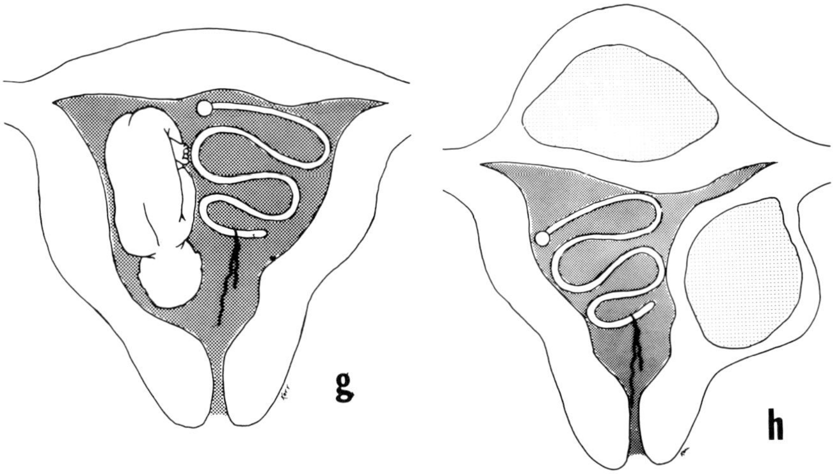

Figure 7.1 Causes of absent IUD tail: (a) absent tail; (b) short tail; (c) device rotation; (d) polar change; (e) incomplete extrusion; (f) complete extrusion; (g) uterine enlargement due to pregnancy and (h) uterine enlargement due to tumor

(Tietze, 1966; Ratnam and Yin, 1968; Hall, 1967; Mishell, 1974). This diagnosis is usually made when the tail of the device is not seen on vaginal examination. Absence of a protruding tail, however, does not necessarily indicate intra-abdominal displacement of the IUD as certain other conditions may also cause the IUD string not to be visible (Table 7.1; Figure 7.1). We believe that conditions enumerated in Table 7.1 occur more often than is generally appreciated.

DIAGNOSIS

Regardless of the location of the device (intrauterine *vs.* extrauterine), whenever the tail is not visible on vaginal examination it is necessary to identify the exact location of the device in order to: (1) avoid an unwanted pregnancy; (2) recommend its removal if within the abdominal cavity; (3) inform the patient of the IUD's status; and (4) prevent potential complications (Baker, 1969; Leventhal *et al.* 1971; Scott, 1968; Swartz, 1970).

To identify the device with missing tail, various procedures outlined in Table 7.1 are recommended. Diagnosis of an intra-abdominally displaced IUD is easily established by a simple flat plate of the abdomen when the device is outside the pelvic cavity. This simple radiologic procedure, however, may fail to differentiate between an intrauterine and extrauterine device when the device is within the confines of the pelvic cavity. To determine the exact location of such a device, it may be necessary to resort to other special diagnostic procedures such as.hysterosalpingography (Dhall *et al.*, 1969), pelvic pneumography (Ansari and Arronet, 1966), and ultrasonography (Ianniruberto and Mastroberodino, 1972; Piiroinen, 1972) (Figure 7.2).

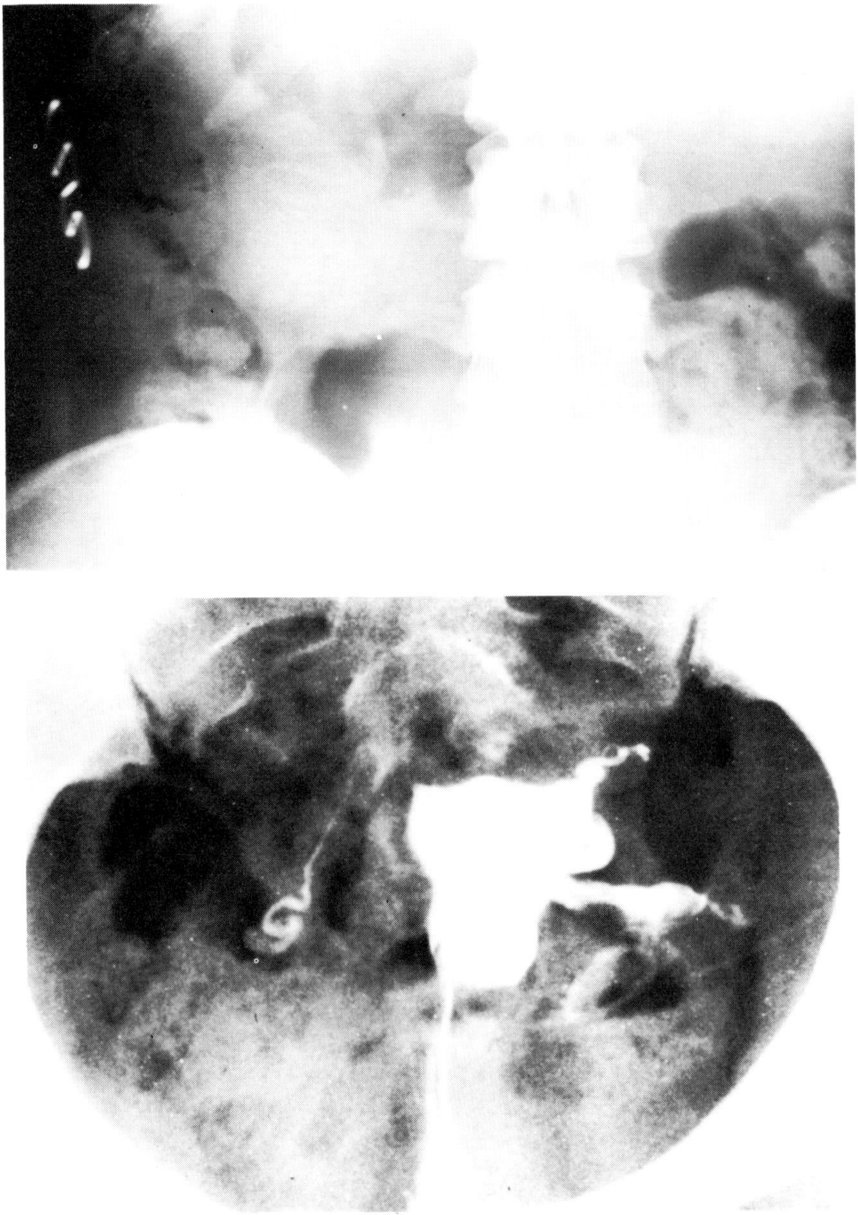

Figure 7.2 Diagnostic procedures for identification of IUD with missing tail. (a) Flat plate of the abdomen showing the IUD outside the pelvic cavity. (b) Hysterosalpingogram showing the IUD (arrow) outside the uterus. (c) Pelvic pneumogram showing IUD inside the uterine cavity; cause for absent tail – uterine enlargement due to fibroid (shown by arrow). (From Ansari, A. H. (1974). *Obstet. Gynecol.*, **44**, 727). (d) Pelvic ultrasound showing intrauterine location of IUD

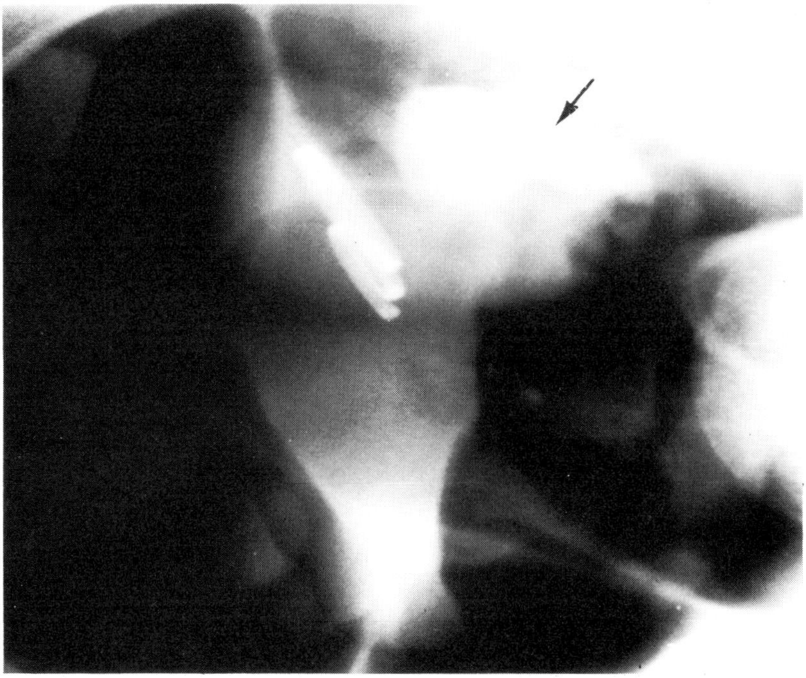

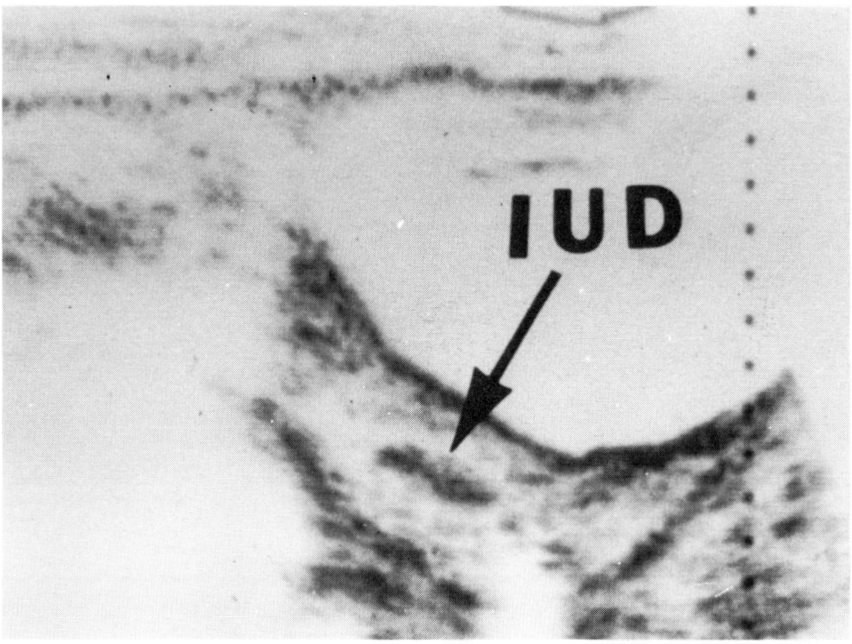
IUD

Occasionally, lateral uterine displacement using a uterine dilator under fluoroscopic observation may be the only means of establishing the exact location of the IUD with a missing tail (Ansari, 1974).

MANAGEMENT

Although removal of a device with missing tail from the uterine cavity is optional and depends on the decision of the patient and her physician, removal is mandatory whenever the device is displaced intra-abdominally.

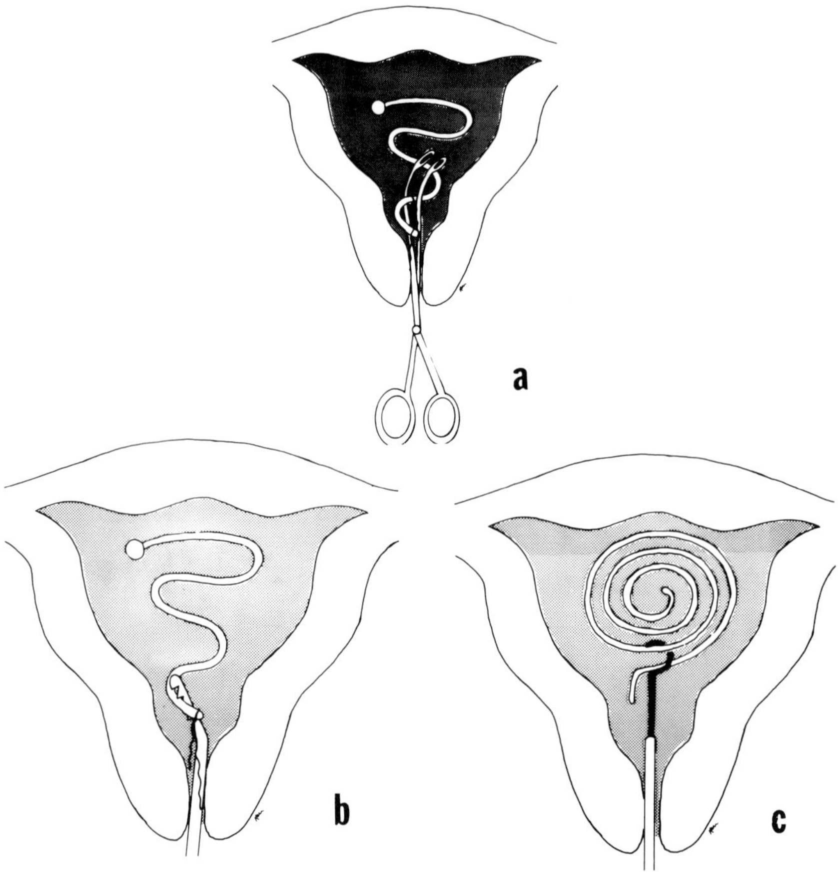

Figure 7.3 Recommended techniques for retrieval of occult IUD: (a) forceps; (b) curette; (c) hook

INTRAUTERINE IUD (OCCULT IUD)

For removal of an IUD with missing tail from the uterine cavity (occult IUD), various methods outlined in Table 7.1 and illustrated in Figure 7.3 have been recommended with varying success (Ansari, 1974; Diakonis and

Weiner, 1974; Shapiro, 1977; Abramovici and Brandes, 1978).

Using a specially designed plastic instrument (MI-Mark, Figure 7.4), we have been able to retrieve several occult IUDs successfully (Ansari and Hoffman, 1981). This is accomplished in most cases with the least amount of discomfort to the patient. Furthermore, application of the cervical tenaculum may not be necessary in many cases, which avoids cervical trauma. The methodology consists of forward progression of the MI-Mark instrument into the uterine cavity by constant and gentle clockwise rotation. Advancement of the MI-Mark through clockwise rotation into the uterine cavity in sufficient length (predetermined by uterine sounding) will usually result in wrapping the tail or a portion of the device around the instrument (Figure 7.5). Withdrawal of the MI-Mark from the uterus while maintaining

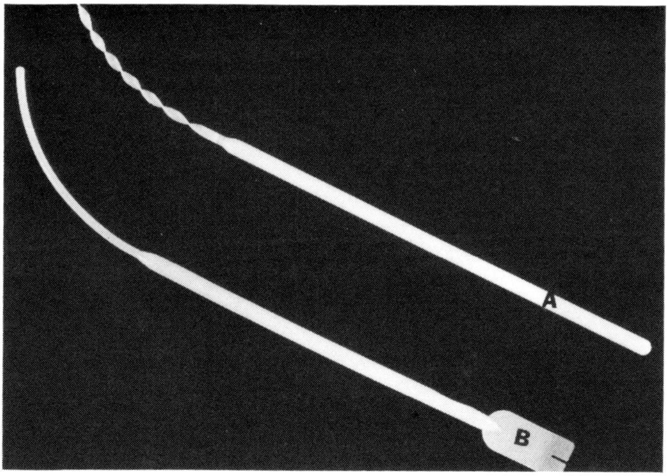

Figure 7.4 MI-Mark instrument: (a) uterine sound; (b) spiral device

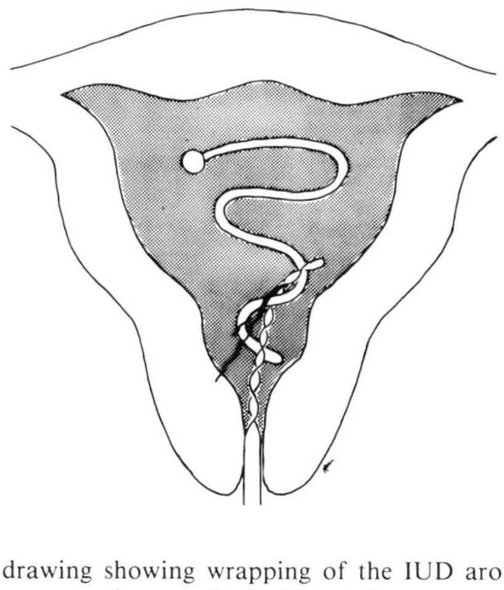

Figure 7.5 Schematic drawing showing wrapping of the IUD around the MI-Mark spiral through clockwise rotation

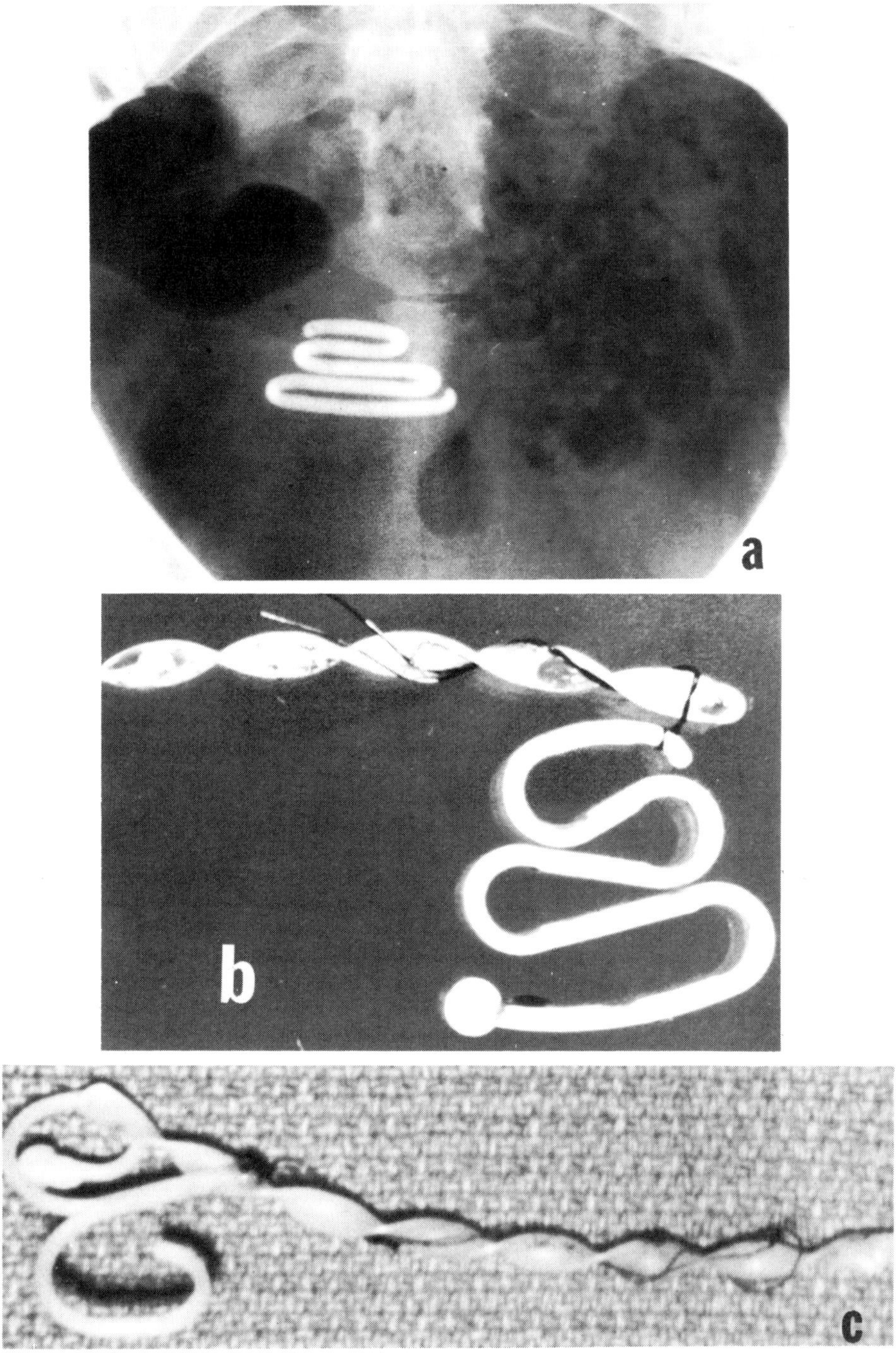

Figure 7.6 Retrieval of occult IUDs using MI-Mark: (a) an occult IUD as the result of polar change; (b) retrieval of the same IUD, (c) retrieval of an occult Saf-T coil

clockwise rotation will therefore result in either retrieval of the tail or the IUD itself (Figure 7.6).

In cases of IUDs partially embedded within the uterine wall, hysteroscopy may be the only successful approach to recovery and should be exercised by an experienced physician (Seigler and Kemmann, 1975; Valle *et al.*, 1977).

INTRA-ABDOMINAL IUD (DISPLACED IUD)

Removal of an intra-abdominally displaced IUD may be accomplished by laparoscopy, laparotomy, colpotomy or culdoscopy (Amman, 1968; Ragab and Sammour, 1969; Smith, 1969; Taylor, 1970). Selection of a particular procedure depends mainly on such factors as location, associated pathology (adhesion, uterine or adnexal pathology requiring corrective surgery), and the experience of the operator. In general, the ultimate decision to remove the device via laparoscope or by means of an abdominal laparotomy depends on the laparoscopic findings.

CONCLUDING REMARKS

Failure to identify the tail of the IUD on speculum examination demands identification of the device location. This is mainly to avoid an unwanted pregnancy and potential complications. In general, removal of an IUD with missing tail may not be necessary when the device is within the uterine cavity (occult IUD). However, removal is indicated in such circumstances as desire for pregnancy, replacement with a new device, particularly in the case of medicated IUD, and associated complications (bleeding, infection, pain, and cramping).

Retrieval of a device with missing tail from the uterine cavity is best accomplished using the MI-Mark instrument. Retrieval is performed as a simple office procedure with minimal trauma and least discomfort. Removal, using other techniques such as hook, forceps, and curette, are both painful and traumatic and very often non-productive.

Dilatation and curettage, a commonly performed procedure for retrieval of an occult IUD, is potentially hazardous and is relatively expensive. Similarly, hysteroscopic removal not only requires special instruments and technical expertise but may also require the use of general anesthesia with its associated hazard and expenses.

An intra-abdominally displaced device should be removed in order to avoid potential complications. This may be accomplished by laparoscopy, laparotomy, culdoscopy, or colpotomy, depending upon location of the device.

References

Abramovici, H. and Brandes, J. M. (1978). A simple ambulatory method for removal of occult IUDs. *Int. J. Fertil.*, **23**, 79

Amman, M. (1968). Colpotomy to retrieve IUD. *Obstet. Gynecol.*, **32**, 294

Ansari, A. H. (1974). Diagnosis and management of intrauterine device with missing tail. *Obstet. Gynecol.*, **44**, 727

Ansari, A. H. and Arronet, G. H. (1966). Pneumo-hysterosalpingography in infertility and related gynecologic conditions. The Foley catheter technique. *Fertil. Steril.*, **17**, 442

Ansari, A. H. and Hoffman, D. (1981). Retrieval of IUD with missing tail using a plastic spiral curette (MI-Mark). *Am. J. Obstet. Gynecol.* (in press)

Baker, J. W. (1969). Serious complications of intrauterine contraceptive devices. *Med. J. Aust.*, **1**, 1126

Dhall, K., Dhall, G. I. and Gupta, B. B. (1969). Uterine perforation with Lippes loop: Detection by hysterography. *Obstet. Gynecol.*, **34**, 226

Diakonis, F. N. and Weiner, C. (1974). Intrauterine device extraction. Safe method utilizing fluoroscopy. *Radiology*, **111**, 479

Hall, R. E. (1967). A reappraisal of intrauterine contraceptive devices. *Am. J. Obstet. Gynecol.*, **99**, 808

Ianniruberto, A. and Mastroberodino, A. (1972). Ultrasonic localization of the Lippes loop. *Am. J. Obstet. Gynecol.*, **114**, 78

Leventhal, J. M., Simon, L. R. and Shpiro, S. S. (1971). Laparoscopic removal of intrauterine contraceptive devices following uterine perforation. *Am. J. Obstet. Gynecol.*, **111**, 102

Mishell, D. R. (1974). Current concepts in contraception. *Clin. Obstet. Gynecol.*, **17**, 35

Piiroinen, O. (1972). Ultrasonic localization of intrauterine contraceptive devices. *Acta Obstet. Gynecol. Scand.*, **51**, 203

Ragab, M. I. and Sammour, M. B. (1969). Sociomedical studies on 60,000 applications for family planning. *Am. J. Obstet. Gynecol.*, **105**, 156

Ratnam, S. S. and Yin, J. C. (1968). Translocation of Lippes loop (The missing loop). *Br. Med J.*, **1**, 612

Scott, R. B. (1968). Critical illnesses and death associated with intrauterine devices. *Obstet. Gynecol.*, **31**, 322

Seigler, A. M. and Kemmann, E. (1974). Hysteroscopic removal of occult intrauterine contraceptive devices. *Obstet. Gynaecol.*, **46**, 604

Shapiro, A. G. (1977). Management of the lost intrauterine contraceptive device. *Obstet. Gynaecol.*, **49**, 238

Smith, D. C. (1969). Removal of an ectopic IUD through the laparoscope. *Am. J. Obstet. Gynecol.*, **105**, 285

Swartz, F. G. (1970). Richter's hernia resulting from displaced intrauterine contraceptive device. *Am. J. Surg.*, **36**, 502

Taylor, M. B. (1970). Operative laparoscopy. *Obstet. Gynecol.*, **35**, 981

Tietze, C. (1966). Contraceptive with intrauterine devices 1959–1966. *Am. J. Obstet. Gynecol.*, **96**, 1042

Valle, R. F., Sciarra, J. J. and Freeman, D. W. (1977) Hysteroscopic removal of intrauterine devices with missing filaments. *Obstet. Gynecol.*, **49**, 55

8
Effect of IUDs on subsequent fertility

K. S. MOGHISSI

Approximately 50–60 million women world-wide are believed to have IUDs. Despite their undisputed safety, IUDs are known to be associated with some troublesome side-effects such as increased bleeding and cramping, and occasional serious and even fatal complications. Numerous publications have dealt with various complications arising from the use of an IUD. Only a few studies have appeared on the effect of the IUD on subsequent fertility. The purpose of this paper is to review the available information on the relationship between the use of an IUD and infertility.

Several studies have indicated that the IUD has no effect on subsequent fertility (Segal and Tietze, 1971; Tietze and Lewit, 1970). More recent reports suggest that the longer a woman uses an IUD, the less her chances relative to non-users of the same age group of conceiving after she dis-

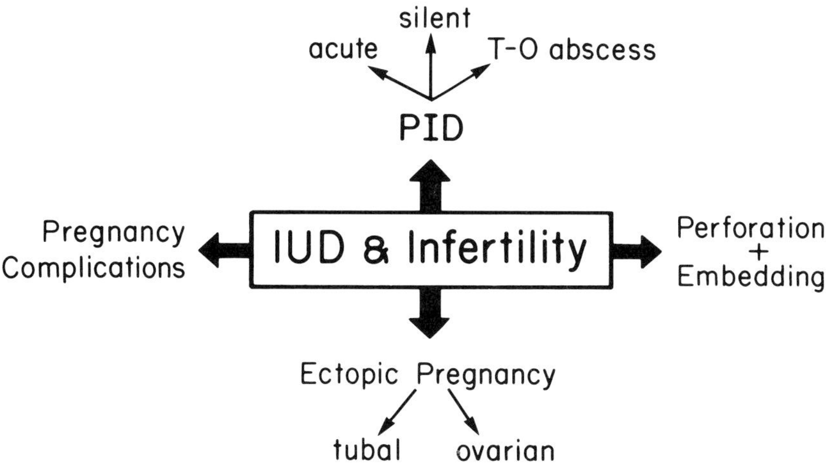

Figure 8.1 IUD complications causing infertility

continues the method (Jain and Moots, 1977). A British study conducted by Vessey *et al.* (1974) has shown that 48.5% of 258 women who had their devices removed to become pregnant had not given birth after 12 months as compared with 29.4% of 1085 women abandoning diaphragms or other traditional contraceptive methods. After 3½ years, however, the difference in the incidence of pregnancies between the two groups had disappeared.

Several IUD complications have the potential of causing infertility. These include pelvic inflammatory disease (PID), ectopic pregnancy, increased incidence of septic abortion when intrauterine pregnancy occurs in the presence of an IUD, and, to a lesser extent, uterine perforation and myometrial embedding (Figure 8.1).

PELVIC INFLAMMATORY DISEASE

Numerous studies have shown that IUD users run a higher risk of PID than non-users. The increased risk begins with the insertion of the IUD and continues as long as the device is in place. Young, nulliparous women who use an IUD are particularly susceptible to PID. As shown in Table 8.1, increased relative risk of PID in IUD users has been found to range from 2.9 (Westrom *et al.*, 1976) to 9.3 (Targum and Wright, 1974).

Table 8.1 Controlled epidemiologic studies of the association between IUDs and PID

Authors	*Type of study*	*No. of subjects*	*RR*
Wright and Laemmle (1968)	Descriptive	108	4.2
Targum and Wright (1974)	Prospective	150	9.3
Faulkner and Ory (1976)	Prospective case-control	250	5.1
Westrom *et al.* (1976)	" "	1 256	2.9
Vessey *et al.* (1976)	Prospective cohort	17 032	3.5
Eschenbach *et al.* (1977)	Prospective case-control	346	4.4

RR = Relative risk

In the USA, Faulkner and Ory (1976), using a prospective case-control design with strict criteria for PID diagnosis, demonstrated that IUD users had 5.1 times the risk of PID as non-users. The fivefold increased risk was present for each 5-year age group, including teenagers. The authors ruled out the possibility of physician ascertainment bias by stratifying the case definition for PID according to subjective and objective parameters; adding the requirement of a temperature of at least 38°C to the case definition increased the relative risk from 2.7 for the less strictly defined cases to 5.1 for those more strictly defined. Moreover, controlling for the frequency of intercourse and the number of sexual partners did not alter the range of this relative risk.

Vessey *et al.* (1976), in a large prospective cohort study of 17 000 contraceptive users from Oxford, UK, have reported that oral contraceptive and diaphragm users had an incidence rate of first presentation for PID of 0.57 per 1000 women-years; IUD users had a rate of 2.02. This 3.5-fold higher relative risk for IUD users was statistically significant and was not due to differences in age, parity, social class, or smoking habits.

In another case–control study of matched pairs, Eschenbach *et al.* (1976) found that the risk of acute PID was 4.4 times higher in IUD users than in non-users. This difference was highly significant. The authors estimated that of approximately 500 000 cases of acute PID occurring annually in the United States an estimated 110 000 are attributable to IUDs. In addition to common pelvic infection such as gonococcal salpingitis and endometritis, some unusual types of PID – e.g. unilateral salpingitis or salpingo-oophoritis (Taylor *et al.*, 1975; Dawood and Birnbaum 1975) and actinomycosis infections (Schiffer *et al.*, 1978) – have been encountered in IUD users.

Nulligravid women who use IUDs seem to be at higher risk of developing PID than women who have been previously pregnant (Eschenbach *et al.*, 1976). Westrom *et al.* (1976) found a 6.9 times increased risk of PID among nulligravid IUD users and 1.7 times increased risk among previously gravid IUD users. The conclusion to be drawn from these studies is that the use of an IUD is associated with a higher risk of PID and the risk is greater in the nulliparous compared with the multiparous woman. Inflammatory diseases of the fallopian tubes lead commonly to subfertility and infertility.

ECTOPIC PREGNANCY

In the USA and UK ectopic pregnancy accounts for approximately 10% of maternal deaths (Beral, 1975; Schneider *et al.*, 1977). More commonly, the ectopic pregnancy compromises the fertility of the affected woman. In studies of IUD users the proportion of pregnancies that are ectopic has varied from less than 1% to more than 25% (Tatum and Schmidt, 1977; Vessey *et al.*, 1974). Most are in the range of 1–5% (Piotrow *et al.*, 1979). By comparison, most studies in western countries indicate proportions of ectopic pregnancies to deliveries in hospital to be near, or below, 1%. For IUD users the chance that a pregnancy will be ectopic has been estimated to be roughly 7–10 times higher than for a non-user, or approximately one in 30 as compared with one in 250 pregnancies of non-IUD users (Piotrow *et al.*, 1979).

Two hypotheses have been advanced to explain the high ratio of ectopic to intrauterine pregnancies in IUD users: (1) IUDs may not prevent ectopic pregnancies as well as they prevent uterine pregnancies; and (2) IUD-related salpingitis may interfere with the transport of a fertilized ovum, making an ectopic pregnancy more likely. While these hypotheses are not mutually exclusive the relative roles they might play would affect the incidence of ectopic pregnancy in IUD users. Ledfeldt *et al.* (1970) estimated that IUDs reduced uterine implantation by 99.5%, tubal implantation by 95%, and ovarian implantation not at all. In support of this hypothesis, it should be noted that in the USA as well as in several other countries there has been a steady rise in the rate of ectopic pregnancies in the last decade (Smith, 1976). Between 1971 and 1977 alone, the rate of ectopic pregnancies according to Curran (1980) doubled from 4.77 per 1000 live births to 9.35 per 1000. Half of these ectopic pregnancies were attributed to tubal disease after PID. Similarly, an increase of 25% in Canada, 24% in England and Wales, and 44% in the Netherlands has been documented.

Another interesting observation is common reports of ovarian pregnancies in association with IUD use. Primary ovarian pregnancy is one of the rarest types of ectopic pregnancies and occurs about one in every 40 000 deliveries with a ratio of 0.7 ovarian per 100 ectopic pregnancies (Ledfeldt *et al.*, 1970). On the other hand, in IUD users a ratio of one ovarian to nine ectopic pregnancies has been observed (Tietze, 1966). Tatum and Schmidt (1977) have recently challenged the Ledfeldt–Tietze hypothesis. They have argued that the risk of ectopic pregnancy rises with age and is higher for women with a history of ectopic pregnancy or of pelvic infection. Also, an increase in the ratio of ectopic to uterine pregnancies with increasing duration of IUD use is known to occur (Jain, 1977; Tatum and Schmidt, 1977; Tatum, 1977, Vessey *et al.*, 1974). Because uterine pregnancy rates decline with duration of IUD use while at the same time the risk of ectopic pregnancy increases with age, ratios of ectopic to uterine pregnancies would be expected to increase over time in any case.

However, the apparent duration of use effect cannot be considered clear evidence for a cause-and-effect relationship, because the highly fertile will become pregnant early in the study, leaving an increasing proportion of subfertile women and women with PID who may be at greater risk for ectopic pregnancy. All of the above indicate that there is a causal relationship between the use of an IUD and the occurrence of ectopic pregnancy. There is no unanimity of opinion as to how this is effected. Most tubal pregnancies are treated by performing a salpingectomy. The effect of an ectopic pregnancy, therefore, on fertility is unquestionable. Repeated extrauterine pregnancies may lead to complete sterility.

PREGNANCY COMPLICATIONS

Approximately 50% of unplanned pregnancies which occur while an IUD is *in utero* will terminate by spontaneous abortion if the IUD is allowed to remain in the uterus (Lewit, 1970; Shine and Thompson, 1974; Vessey *et al.*, 1974). This is 3–5 times the incidence of abortion observed in the general population. Removing the IUD will reduce the risks of spontaneous abortion by at least one half. Continued presence of an IUD in a pregnant uterus may also cause premature rupture of membranes (Dreishpoon, 1975). The risk of sepsis associated with accidental pregnancy in IUD users is considerable. Septic abortion and even death have been encountered in these patients (Christian, 1974).

In 31 consecutive pregnant women with IUD *in situ*, Dreishpoon (1975) observed three cases of septic abortion and one case of amnionitis due to premature rupture of membrane. Similarly, a survey of US physicians by the United States Food and Drug Administration uncovered 289 cases of septic mid-trimester abortion in IUD users, including 21 deaths (Jennings, 1974).

Clearly, septic abortion and chorioamnionitis, even when treated, would impair future fertility. Although precise data are not available, one could assume that severe endometritis and/or salpingo-oophoritis, particularly when associated with abscess formation, would lead to tubal obstruction which may necessitate salpingectomy and even hysterectomy.

UTERINE PERFORATION AND MYOMETRIAL EMBEDDING

Two types of perforation have been described: fundal and cervical. The risk of perforation depends on the size, shape, and consistency of the device, on the technique of insertion, on the status and configuration of the uterus, and above all on the skill and experience of the operator (Tatum, 1977). The incidence of perforation is difficult to establish. The cooperative statistical program estimated the incidence of perforation at less than 1 or 2 per 1000 insertions (Tietze and Lewit, 1970). Mishell (1974) has indicated a range from 1/350 to 1/2500 insertions.

Cervical perforation has particularly been observed with Copper-7 but may be seen with other IUDs. Perforations are usually asymptomatic and only rarely cause the loss of reproductive function. Once the IUD has been retrieved no lasting effect is expected to occur. Embedding may lead to a reduction in contraceptive efficacy and subsequent pregnancy, abortion, and possible sepsis. Embedding may also be associated with difficult removal of the IUD, necessitating surgical interventions which may occasionally impair fertility.

CONCLUDING REMARKS

Despite their undisputed effectiveness and safety, the IUDs have the potential of impairing subsequent fertility by their ability to cause perforation, embedding, and a higher rate of PID, ectopic pregnancy, and septic abortion (Figure 8.1). These risks can be minimized by proper selection of candidates for insertion of an IUD and prompt recognition and management of the complications. Based on current data, I believe that the IUDs should rarely if ever be inserted in young nulligravid women, particularly those with small uteri. Oral contraceptives rather than IUDs are best suited to these women. Oral contraceptives should also be considered in preference to IUD for sexually active females with multiple sexual partners who are at high risk for PID.

Patients should be adequately counseled regarding the symptoms of pelvic infection and ectopic pregnancies and warned of pregnancy complications in the presence of an IUD. The IUD should be removed as soon as a pregnancy is diagnosed in an IUD wearer. If the IUD cannot be retrieved, termination of pregnancy should be offered to the patient. Patients who refuse therapeutic abortion must be carefully followed up. All pelvic infections should be vigorously treated with removal of the IUD and appropriate antibiotic and supportive therapy.

Suspected cases of ectopic pregnancies should be carefully evaluated and, if necessary, subjected to diagnostic laparoscopy. These measures would undoubtedly enhance the safety of IUDs, increase their appeal, and minimize their deleterious effect on the patient's future fertility.

References

Beral, V. (1975). An epidemiological study of recent trends in ectopic pregnancy. *Br. J. Obstet. Gynaecol.*, **82**, 775

Christian, C. D. (1974). Maternal deaths associated with an intrauterine device. *Am. J. Obstet. Gynecol.*, **119**, 441

Curran, J. (1980). Rates of ectopic pregnancy, sterility following PID rise. *Contracept. Technol. Update.*, **1**, 17

Dawood, M. Y. and Birnbaum, S. J. (1975). Unilateral tubo-ovarian abscess and intrauterine contraceptive device. *Obstet. Gynecol.*, **46**, 429

Dreishpoon, I. H. (1975). Complications of pregnancy with an intrauterine contraceptive device in situ. *Am. J. Obsetet. Gynecol.*, **121**, 412

Eschenbach, D. A., Harnisch, J. P. and Holmes, K. K. (1977). Pathogenesis of acute pelvic inflammatory disease: role of contraception and other factors. *Am. J. Obstet. Gynecol.*, **128**, 838

Faulkner, W. L. and Ory, H. W. (1976). Intrauterine devices and acute pelvic inflammatory disease. *J. Am. Med. Assoc.*, **235**, 1851

Jain, A. K. (1977). Nonmedicated intrauterine devices: review and assessment. In *World Health Organization Regulation of Human Fertility*, p. 361. (Copenhagen: Scriptor)

Jain, A. K. and Moots, B. (1977). Fecundability following the discontinuation of IUD use among Taiwanese women. *J. Biol. Sci.*, **9**, 135

Jennings, J. (1974). *Report of Safety and Efficacy of Dalkon Shield and Other IUDs*, p. 19 (New York: FDA Ad Hoc Obstetrics and Gynecology Advisory Committee)

Ledfeldt, H., Tietze, C. and Gorstein, F. (1970). Ovarian pregnancy and the intrauterine device. *Am. J. Obstet. Gynecol.*, **108**, 1005

Lewit, S. (1970). Outcome of pregnancy with intrauterine devices. *Contraception*, **2**, 2

Lippes, J. (1975). Infection and the IUD. A preliminary report. *Contraception*, **12**, 103

Mishell, D. R. (1974). Current concepts in contraception. *Clin. Obstet. Gynecol.*, **17**, 35

Piotrow, P. T., Rinehart, W. and Schmidt, J. C. (1979). IUD update on safety, effectiveness and research. *Population Reports*, **7**, 50 (series B, no. 3)

Schiffer, M. A., Elquezabal, A. and Allen, A. C. (1978). Actinomycosis infections associated with intrauterine contraceptive device and a vaginal pessary. *Adv. Planned Parenthood*, **12**, 183

Schneider, J., Berger, C. J. and Cattell, C. (1977) Maternal mortality due to ectopic pregnancy. A review of 102 deaths. *Obstet. Gynecol.*, **49**, 557

Segal, S. J. and Tietze, C. (1971). Contraceptive technology. Current and prospective methods. *Rep. Pop. Fam. Plann.*, **1**, 1

Shine, R. M. and Thompson, J. F. (1974) The in situ IUD and pregnancy outcome. *Am. J. Obstet. Gynecol.*, **119**, 124

Smith, D. (1976). *Abortion Surveillance.* DHEW Publication No: (CDC) 78-8205. (Rockville, Md: National Center for Health Statistics, hospital discharge survey)

Targum, S. D. and Wright, N. H. (1974). Association of the intrauterine device and pelvic inflammatory disease: a retrospective pilot study. *Am. J. Epidemiol.*, **100**. 262

Tatum, H. J. (1977). Clinical aspects of intrauterine contraception. *Fertil. Steril.*, **28**, 3

Tatum, H. J. and Schmidt, F. H. (1977). Contraceptive and sterilization practices and extrauterine pregnancy: a realistic perspective. *Fertil. Steril.*, **28**, 407

Taylor, E. S., McMillan, J. H., Greer, B. E., Droegemuller, W. and Thompson, H. E. (1975). The intrauterine device and tubo-ovarian abscess. *Am. J. Obstet. Gynecol.*, **123**, 338

Tietze, C. (1966). Contraception with intrauterine devices. *Am. J. Obstet. Gynecol.*, **96**, 1043

Tietze, C. and Lewit, S. (1970). Evaluation of intrauterine devices: ninth progress report of the cooperative statistical program. *Stud. Family Planning*, **55**, 1

Vessey, M. P., Johnson, B., Doll, R. and Peto, R. (1974). Outcome of pregnancy in women using an intrauterine device. *Lancet*, **1**, 495

Vessey, M., Doll, R., Peto, R., Johnson, B. and Wiggins, P. (1976). A longterm followup study of women using different methods of contraception. An interim report. *J. Biosoc. Sci.*, **8**, 373

Westrom, L., Bengtsson, L. P. and Mardh, P. A. (1976). The risk of pelvic inflammatory disease in women using intrauterine contraceptive devices as compared to nonusers. *Lancet*, **2**, 221

Wright, N. H. and Laemmle, P. (1968). Acute pelvic inflammatory disease in an indigent population: an estimate of its incidence and relationship to the methods of contraception. *Am. J. Obstet. Gynecol.*, **101**, 979

9
Fertility control in women aged 35 years and older: the role of intrauterine steroidal contraception

M. ROBINSON AND Y. GIBOR

Today's woman over age 35 has different problems in selecting a contraceptive than her counterpart had 10 years ago (Table 9.1). A woman who was over 35 in 1970, for instance, usually started her sexually active life with only a limited ability to control predictable fertility independent from her partner. Planning life goals was uncertain because of the assumed inevitability of pregnancy. Her 'on-again-off-again' participation in the workforce often kept her from being considered for prime employment. The married over-35 woman of 1970, however, had usually completed her childbearing plans, had little awareness of the risks of oral contraceptives (OCs), and had ordinarily been a user at one time of a coitus-related contraceptive. For all these reasons, the 1970s over-35 contraceptor was usually amenable to continued use of the pill or diaphragm (or a return to the latter), or was a candidate for sterilization.

Today's over-35 woman presents a different picture, because she is at less risk from unplanned childbearing. Early in their reproductive life, these women usually assume independent control over their fertility – through OC or IUD use. This control has given many options in both personal and professional life.

Table 9.1 Changing characteristics over one decade in women over the age of 35

Characteristic	*1970s*	*1980s*
Control over life and fertility	Limited	Most women have had – and will continue to need – control because of sexual activity, inflationary pressures, and career expectations
Prior use of effective contraceptives (OC, IUD)	Limited	Most have used effective contraceptives during the past decade
Childbearing	Usually completed	Many postpone having children, and some remarry and want more children
Awareness of risks associated with OCs	Steadily increasing	

Planning career goals is relatively unobstructed by unplanned pregnancies or the fear of such pregnancies. For these reasons - or because of a second marriage - women may plan a pregnancy later in life than women of the previous decade. Inflationary pressures or the desire for professional advancement, or other social factors, may control reproductive life. The woman of the 1980s needs a reliable, safe, and reversible contraceptive.

Unfortunately, as a woman approaches 35, her contraceptive options diminish. Oral contraceptives lose favor because of age-related risk factors; excessive menstrual bleeding may rule out use of an unmedicated or copper IUD. Yet prior use of convenient contraceptives may diminish the woman's acceptance of methods that require motivation from her partner or compliance at each sexual encounter. The rise in incidence of sterilization and in the use of barrier methods is perhaps more reflective of limited choice than of preference. For this group of women, intrauterine steroidal contraception may offer an especially attractive alternative to other methods.

INTRAUTERINE CONTRACEPTION WITH PROGESTERONE

The concept of continuous intrauterine administration of progesterone, as originally presented (Scommegna, 1972), is based on four observations:

(1) The estrogenic component of oral contraceptives is not essential for contraception.
(2) Progestin-only mini-pills provide adequate contraception without inhibiting ovulation.
(3) The mini-pill interferes with nidation and may change the cervical mucus, thus preventing sperm penetration.
(4) Most contraceptive failures associated with the mini-pill relate to poor patient compliance.

Continuous intrauterine administration of low doses of progesterone may therefore provide effective contraception. Such a method would not require patient compliance and would be unlikely to cause systemic side-effects.

PROGESTASERT INTRAUTERINE PROGESTERONE CONTRACEPTIVE SYSTEM (TIPCS)

Concept

The Progestasert system (Figure 9.1) is a T-shaped (Tatum, 1972), progesterone-containing platform of ethylene/vinyl acetate copolymer that continuously delivers 65 μg/day of progesterone directly to the uterine lumen for one year (Figure 9.2). Suppression of the endometrium is the system's only detectable pharmacologic action; studies with prototype systems releasing 5–110 μg/day of progesterone showed that the 65 μg/day release rate maximized this action.

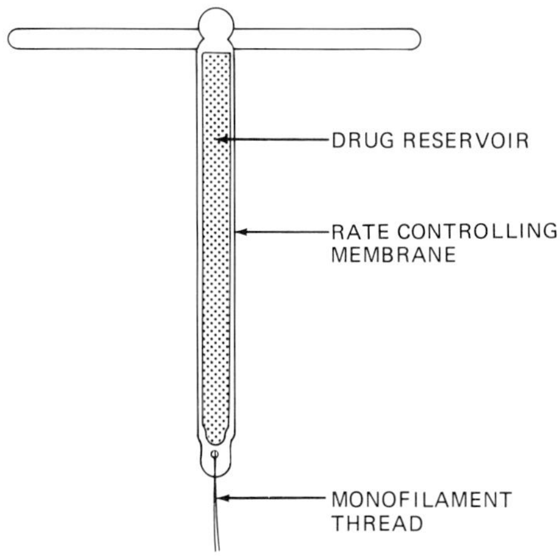

Figure 9.1 Diagram of the Progestasert intrauterine progesterone contraceptive system

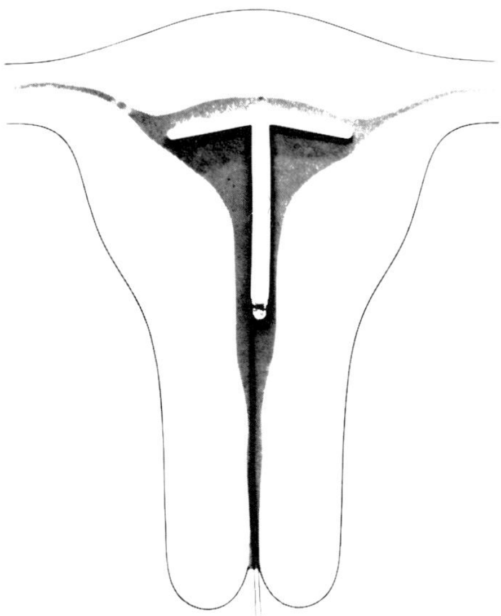

Figure 9.2 Representation of the Progestasert system in the uterus

Database

Experience with the Progestasert system is based on 130 966 woman-months of use in 7651 women (12 102 insertions). Of these women, 886 were older than 35. Clinical trials were conducted in more than 40 centers worldwide, and included patients from both public health clinics and private practices. Exclusion criteria included: existing pelvic inflammatory disease (PID) or a history of chronic episodes of such infections; reproductive tract malignancy; or anatomic abnormalities preventing effective placement of the system. Concomitant use of other contraceptive methods was not permitted.

Effectiveness in women over age 35

Phase III clinical data were pooled and analyzed by the life table method (Tietze and Lewit, 1973). Pregnancy, expulsions, and medical removals were considered use-related discontinuations. Scheduled removals, releases from study, and lost to follow-up (LFU) were considered non-use-related and were ignored in continuation rate calculations. Table 9.2 shows the life table cumulative rates of major events for Progestasert system users aged 35 and older (through 12 months of use). For this population, life table rates are significantly lower than event rates reported for IUDs in general.

Table 9.2 Life table rates during Progestasert system use in women aged over 35 (12 months of use)

Event	*Rate*
Pregnancy	1.1 ± 0.4
Expulsion	2.3 ± 0.5
Removal	
Medical	7.2 ± 1.3
Non-medical	1.3 ± 0.4
Continuation (%)	88.1 ± 1.1
Woman-months	10 100
No. of women	886
Lost to follow-up	11.8 ± 1.1

LIFE RISK TO WOMEN OVER AGE 35: OTHER CONTRACEPTIVES *VS*. THE PROGESTASERT SYSTEM

Since no Progestasert-system-related deaths have been reported, the theoretical life risk for women over age 35 who use this device was calculated by the method described in Table 9.3. This method yields life risks of 1.0 and 1.2 per 100 000 women per year for ages 35–39 and for ages 40–44, respectively. When these rates are compared with rates reported (Tietze and Lewit, 1979) for other methods of contraception in these age groups, the risk of death for ages 35–39 is: 1/21 that of non-contracepting women; 1/32 that of oral contraceptive users who smoke; 1/10 that of oral contraceptive users who do not smoke; 1/10 that associated with tubal ligation (Beral, 1979); 1/250–1/60 that associated with hysterectomy (Cole and Berlin, 1977; CPHA, 1976); 1/2 that of IUD users overall; and 1/5 that of barrier method users. For ages 40–44, the ratios are similar except that the risk doubles in oral contraceptive users. In both groups, barrier methods used in conjunction with abortion are somewhat safer than the Progestasert system.

Table 9.3 Calculation of life risk for women aged over 35

Life risk = birth-related risk + method-related risk

$$\text{Birth-related risk/100 000} = \frac{\text{Maternal deaths}}{\text{Births for women aged over } 35^{a}} \times \begin{array}{l}\text{IPCS uterine}\\ \text{pregnancy rate}\\ \text{for women aged}\\ \text{over 35 per 100}\\ \text{woman-years.}\end{array} \times 10^{3}$$

Method-related risk/100 000 = Risk from EP + risk from PID

$$\text{EP risk/100 000} = \frac{\text{Maternal deaths (EP, 1977)}^{b}}{\text{EP (1977)}^{c}} \times \begin{array}{l}\text{IPCS EP rate}\\ \text{for women aged}\\ \text{over 35 per 100}\\ \text{woman-years.}\end{array} \times 10^{3}$$

$$\text{PID risk/100 000} = \frac{\text{Deaths from PID (1975)}^{b}}{\text{No. cases PID (1975)}^{d}} \times \begin{array}{l}\text{IPCS PID rate}\\ \text{for women aged}\\ \text{over 35 per 100}\\ \text{woman-years.}\end{array} \times 10^{3}$$

[a] Tietze and Lewit (1979)
[b] Burnham (unpublished observations, 1979)
[c] Smith (unpublished observations, 1978)
[d] Eschenbach (1976)
EP = Ectopic pregnancy

THERAPEUTIC IMPLICATIONS OF INTRAUTERINE PROGESTERONE FOR WOMEN OVER AGE 35

Effect on bleeding and pain

During Phase III trials, it became clear that the Progestasert system – like

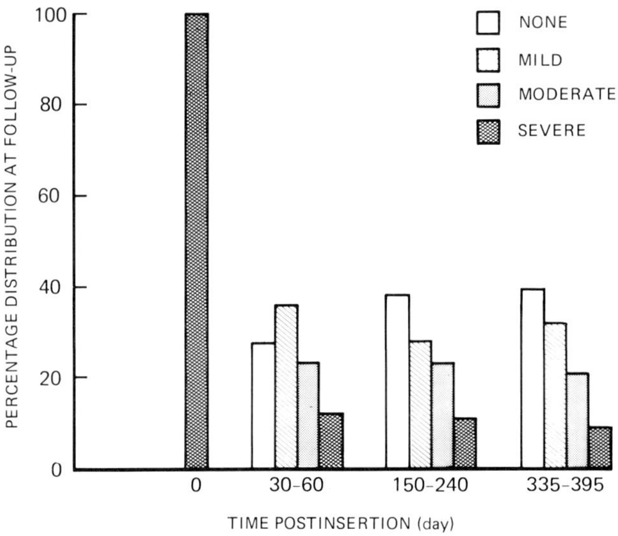

Figure 9.3 Menstrual cramps in 253 women with severe cramps at insertion of the Progestasert system

oral contraceptives, but unlike other IUDs – reduced menstrual blood loss and pain. Women who reported having heavy blood loss upon admission to the study reported a significant reduction 60 days after insertion. Those with severe menstrual cramps upon admission also reported a lessening of their symptoms after insertion (Figure 9.3).

Several quantitative studies of blood loss have shown that while other IUDs increase the amount of blood loss by 50% (e.g. copper IUDs) to 100% (e.g. inert IUDs), progesterone-releasing IUDs decrease bleeding by an average of 50% (Cohen and Gibor, 1980) (Figure 9.4).

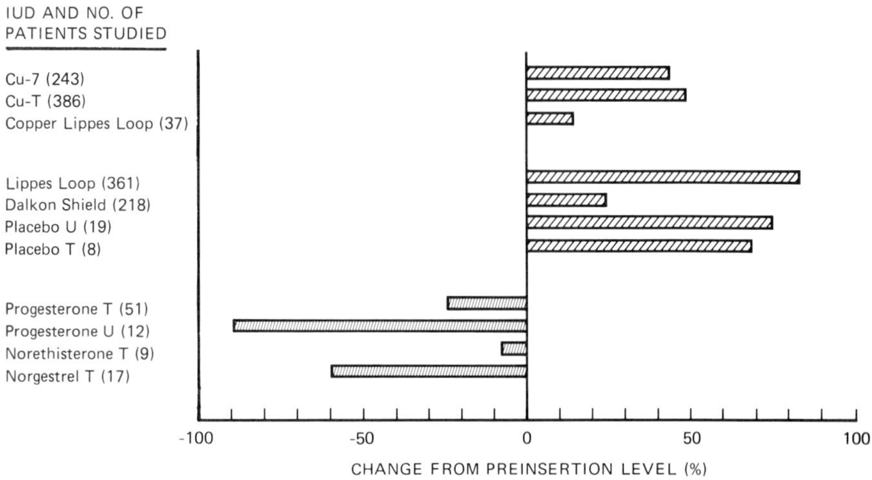

Figure 9.4 Change in menstrual blood loss for various medicated and non-medicated intrauterine devices

In a double-blind comparative trial (data on file at ALZA) patients had insertions of either the Progestasert system or another IUD. In 36 women using the Progestasert system, the average menstrual blood loss – measured before and during several cycles after insertion – *declined* from 40.8 ± 4.6 ml to 20.4 ± 2.7 ml (Table 9.4). For other IUDs, average menstrual blood loss concentrations *rose* from 32.4 ± 4.4 ml preinsertion to 54.5 ± 6.6 ml posinsertion. Thus, in contrast to other IUDs, the Progestasert system reduces volume of menstrual blood loss to about 50% of its preinsertion level.

Table 9.4 Change in menstrual blood loss (MBL) with use of Progestasert system (IPCS) and other IUDs

	No. of women	*Mean (± SE) preinsertion MBL* (ml)	*Mean (± SE) postinsertion MBL* (ml)
IPCS	36	40.8 ± 4.6	20.4 ± 2.7
Other IUDs	32	32.4 ± 4.4	54.5 ± 6.6

Three factors observed during use of the Progestasert system may contribute to the decrease in bleeding and cramps:

(1) Suppression of the endometrium significantly reduces the endometrial hyperemia that is typical of the secretory phase.
(2) Fibrinolytic activity in the endometrium decreases; increased fibrinolytic activity is known to increase menorrhagia during use of other IUDs.
(3) $PGF_{2\alpha}$ concentrations in menstrual blood, which affect blood loss and uterine contractility, also decrease significantly after the Progestasert system is inserted (Trobough *et al.*, 1978; Zahradnik *et al.*, 1978).

The documented effect of exogenous intrauterine progesterone in reducing menstrual bleeding has particular importance to women approaching climacterium. These women often experience excessive menstrual blood loss because of ovulatory failure, unopposed estrogenic effects, and poor luteal function. Among many older women, these symptoms have previously precluded use of IUDs because of their usual effect in increasing menstrual bleeding. Systemically administered hormones also benefit excessive menstrual bleeders, but the Progestasert system avoids systemic hormonal affects and their special risks in older age groups.

Treatment of endometrial pathologies

The incidence of uterine pathology (e.g. dysfunctional uterine bleeding and endometrial hyperplasia) rises in the over-35 age group. These pathologic conditions can result from unopposed estrogen effects on the endometrium. In some cases, they progress to endometrial carcinoma.

The significant anti-estrogenic effect of the Progestasert system in the endometrium, as well as its reduction of bleeding and pain, strongly suggest that it can replace systemic progestins, not only as a contraceptive but also in treatment of some endometrial pathologies.

In a study of eight patients with adenomatous hyperplasia (Basbaum *et al.*, 1978) in which the Progestasert system was used as the only treatment, complete regression of the lesion occurred within 1 year. Thus, women so treated may avoid the need for hysterectomy.

CONCLUDING REMARKS

Assessment of current fertility control methods reveals that most are unsuitable for women over age 35. Women of this age group – particularly those who smoke – should avoid oral contraceptive use (Tietze and Lewit, 1979). Since many women entering this age group have utilized sophisticated contraceptive technology throughout their sexually active lives, techniques that require compliance at each sexual encounter are unappealing. The drawbacks of sterilization, its numerous side-effects, morbidity, and life risks are gaining wider recognition (Athari *et al.*, 1978;

Lauersen, 1979; Chi *et al.*, 1979). Publications (Ringrose, 1974; Radwanska *et al.*, 1979; Chamberlain and Foulkes, 1975) on postoperative alterations in the menstrual pattern, reflecting observed changes in functioning of the pituitary–ovarian axis, suggest an early degeneration of the ovary, probably due to impaired blood supply. This may lead to undesired early menopause. Many patients regret their decision to be sterilized and request reanastomosis. This delicate, time-consuming, and expensive procedure (Hulka, 1978; Lauersen, 1979) has a low success rate and some risk of subsequent morbidity.

A comparison of the Progestasert system with other methods of contraception (Table 9.5) suggests that this device may offer specific advantages as a contraceptive to women aged 35 and over.

Table 9.5 Attributes of the Progestasert system and other methods of contraception for women aged over 35[a]

Benefit	*IPCS*	*OC*	*IUD*	*Barrier*	*Sterilization*
Minimizes systemic effects	+ +	− − −	+ +	+ +	+ +
Counteracts unopposed estrogen	+ +	+ +	0	0	0
Decreases dysfunctional uterine bleeding	+ +	+ +	− − −	0	− −
Provides effective contraception	+ +	+ +	+ +	−	+ + +

[a] Number of plus signs indicates degree of benefit; number of minus signs indicates severity of disadvantages; zero indicates no effect

References

Athari, T. A. and Ravangard, F. (1978). Ectopic pregnancy following tubal sterilizations. *W. Va. Med. J.*, **74**, 229

Basbaum, C., Mattosinho-França, L. C. and Rodrigues de Lima, G. (1978). Local progesterone action on adenomatous hyperplasia: a preliminary report. In Mishell, D. R. and Martínez-Manautou (eds.) *Proceedings of the Symposium on Clinical Experience with the Progesterone Uterine Therapeutic System, Acapulco, Oct. 15–16, 1976*, p. 47. (Amsterdam: Excerpta Medica)

Beral, V. (1979). Reproductive mortality. *Br. Med. J.*, **2**, 632

Chamberlain, G. and Foulkes, J. (1975). Late complications of sterilization by laparoscopy. *Lancet*, **2**, 878

Chi, I.-C., Gardner, S. D. and Laufe, L. E. (1979). The history of pregnancies that occur following female sterilization. *Int. J. Gynecol. Obstet.*, **17**, 265

Cohen, B. J. B. and Gibor, Y. (1980). Anemia and menstrual blood loss. *Obstet. Gynecol. Surv.*, **35**, 597

Cole, P. and Berlin, J. (1977). Elective hysterectomy. *Am. J. Obstet. Gynecol.*, **129**, 117

Commission on Professional and Hospital Activities (1976). *Hospital Mortality: PAS Hospitals, United States, 1972–73*, p. 216. (Ann Arbor, MI: CPHA)

Eschenbach, D. A. (1976). Acute pelvic inflammatory disease: etiology, risk factors and pathogenesis. *Clin. Obstet. Gynecol.*, **19**, 147

Hulka, J. F. (1978). Current status on the reversibility of sterilization. *Res. Reprod.*, **10**, 1

Lauersen, N. (1979). A closer look at sterilization. *Med. World News*, May 28, p. 87

Radwanska, E., Berger, G. S. and Hammond, J. (1979). Luteal deficiency among women with normal menstrual cycles, requesting reversal of tubal sterilization. *Obstet. Gynecol.*, **54**, 189

Ringrose, C. A. D. (1974). Post tubal ligation menorrhagia and pelvic pain. *Int. J. Fertil.*, **19**, 168

Scommegna, A. (1972). Intrauterine administration of progesterone by a slow releasing device. *Fertil. Steril.*, **21**, 201

Tatum, H. J. (1972). Intrauterine contraception. *Am. J. Obstet. Gynecol.*, **112**, 1000

Tietze, C. and Lewit, S. (1973). Recommended procedures for the statistical evaluation of intrauterine contraception. *Stud. Family Planning*, **4**, 35

Tietze, C. and Lewit, S. (1979). Life risks associated with reversible methods of fertility regulation. *Int. J. Gynecol. Obstet.*, **16**, 456

Trobough, G., Guderian, A. M., Erickson, R. R., Tillson, S. A., Leong, P., Swisher, D. A. and Pharriss, B. B. (1978). The effect of exogenous intrauterine progesterone on the amount of prostaglandin $F_{2\alpha}$ content of menstrual blood loss in dysmenorrheic women. *J. Reprod. Med.*, **21**, 153

Zahradnik, H. P., Stengle, E. Kraut, E. and Breckwoldt, M. (1978). [New aspects of pathogenesis and treatment of dysmenorrhea: prostaglandin $F_{2\alpha}$ level in the menstrual blood.] *Dtsch. Med. Wochenschr.*, **103**, 1270 [German]

10
IUD-induced bleeding: complications and management

P. F. TAUBER, J. C. GOODPASTURE, M. NOHLEN AND H. LUDWIG

Excessive uterine hemorrhage associated with intrauterine contraception is common and is the most frequent complication of this contraceptive method (Piotrow *et al.,* 1979). Physicians are therefore quite often presented with the problem of finding effective therapy for IUD-associated hypermenorrhea. The excessive bleeding should be treated in all circumstances, regardless of the individual, geographic and/or ethnological differences in bleeding patterns. In addition to the fact that patients are often worried by the inconvenience of excess bleeding, uterine hemorrhage favors expulsion of the device as well as ascension of bacteria into the upper genital tract. Even more problematic is that anemia may develop, and if already present may be maintained or even become extreme while the IUD is in place. The only effective treatment at present for these IUD-related side-effects is removal of the device. This is often the case even though the hypermenorrhea is most commonly experienced for a limited time span, usually for the first 6 months after insertion. Unfortunately, removal of the device leaves the woman without safe contraceptive protection.

In lesser developed countries where intrauterine contraception has recently gained wide-spread acceptance as a relatively safe and easy-to-use method, physicians and patients must be particularly concerned about both hypermenorrhea and high removal rates. In these countries malnutrition, anemia, consuming infections and parasitic diseases, high parity with short birth-to-birth intervals, and long periods of lactation are part of a 'normal' life, factors which in themselves cause a high mortality rate and low life expectancy. For women in these countries, additional blood loss due to contraception with IUDs is not acceptable, and the IUD becomes an even more unfavorable method of birth control. For these reasons, scientific and clinical efforts have been greatly increased in recent years in an attempt to reduce IUD-associated hypermenorrhea, and thus to increase acceptability of the IUD.

Although various alterations in the shape and design of IUDs for

Table 10.1 Non-hormonal medications for prophylaxis and treatment of uterine bleeding in women

Year(s)	*Author(s)*	*Substance*	*Dosage and route of administration*	*Indication*	*Effect*	*Side-effects*
(I) Synthetic proteinase inhibitors: Mechanism(s) of action – inhibition of plasminogen activation and fibrinolysis						
1965, 1967, 1971	Nilsson *et al.*	EACA	12–18 g/day; oral	Menorrhagia	+	Gastrointestinal complaints
		AMCA	6–24 g/day; oral	Menorrhagia	+	Gastrointestinal complaints
		PAMBA	3–4 g/day; oral	Menorrhagia	+	Gastrointestinal complaints
1965	Ludwig and Mehring	EACA	4–8 g/day; oral, days 2–4	Hypermenorrhea	+	Gastrointestinal complaints
1968	Vermylen *et al.*	EACA	6 × 1 g/day; oral	Menorrhagia	+	Hypotensive reaction
1970	Callender *et al.*	AMCA	4 × 1 g/day; oral, days 1–4	Menorrhagia	+	Headache
1970	Weström and Bengtsson	AMCA	4 × 1.5 g/day; oral, days 1–5	IUD patients	+	Rare, mostly gastrointestinal complaints
1973	MacMath	EACA	4 × 2 g/day; oral	IUD patients	(+)	Nausea
			4 × 3 g/day; oral	IUD patients	+	Nausea
1975	Kasonde and Bonnar	EACA	4 × 3 g/day; oral, days 1–7 or other menstrual days	IUD patients	+	Nausea, dizziness, headache
1975	Tauber and Wolf	AMCA	1–2 g; intrauterine at onset of menses	IUD patients	+	None
1977a, 1978	Tauber *et al.*	EACA	24 mg on Lippes Loop	IUD patients	+	None
1975	Wolf *et al.*	AMCA	2 g; intrauterine	IUD patients	+	None
1976	Ragab and Thomas	AMCA	AMCA-U-Coil	IUD patients	+	None
1977	Hefnawi *et al.*	AMCA	AMCA-Lippes Loop	IUD patients	– (possible technical problem)	None
1977	Lauder and Lauder	EACA	4 × 3 g/day; oral, days 1–4	Hypermenorrhea (some IUD patients)	+	Nausea, headache, dizziness

(II) Natural proteinase inhibitors: Mechanism(s) of action – inhibition of kinin generation and of plasmin						
1975	Wolf *et al.*	Aprotinin	200 000 KIU[a];	IUD patients	+	None
1977b	Tauber *et al.*	Aprotinin	1–2 ml; intrauterine (100 000 KIU/ml)	IUD patients	+ +	None None
1978	Genicot	Aprotinin	100 000 KIU; intrauterine	IUD patients	+	None
(III) Anti-inflammatory drugs: Mechanism of action – prostaglandin synthetase inhibition						
1976	Damarawy and Toppozada	Indomethacin	3 × 25 mg/day; oral, days – 2 to + 2	IUD patients with menorrhagia	+	Gastrointestinal complaints, edema
1976	Anderson *et al.*	Mefenamic acid	3 × 500 mg/day; oral during bleeding	IUD patients with menorrhagia	+	Teratogenic? Increased pregnancy rate?
		Flufenamic acid	3 × 200 mg/day; oral during bleeding	IUD patients with menorrhagia	+	Fertility?
1978	Guillebaud *et al.*	Mefenamic acid	3 × 500 mg oral/day maximum until day 7	IUD patients with hypermenorrhea	+	Headache, indigestion
1978	Ylikorkala *et al.*	Tolfenamic acid	3 × 200 mg/day; oral, days 1–7 after IUD insertion	IUD patients	+	Gastrointestinal complaints
(IV) Synthetic cyclohexadines: Mechanism(s) of action – effect on platelet function, increased capillary resistance, and antihyaluronidase activity						
1975	Kasonde and Bonnar	Ethamsylate	4 × 3 g/day during menstruation	IUD patients	+	Nausea, headache, dizziness
1976	Harrison and Campbell	Ethamsylate	4 × 500 mg/day; days – 5 to + 5	IUD patients	+	Minor, same as placebo group
1978	Kovács and Annus	Ethamsylate	3 × 500 mg/day; days – 4 to + 6	IUD patients	+	Gastrointestinal complaints
(V) Ergotalkaloids: Mechanism(s) of action – vasoconstriction and uterine contraction						
1971	Nilsson and Rybo	Methyl-ergobasein-maleate	0.75 mg/day; oral, days 1–4	Menorrhagia	–	Gastrointestinal complaints

Table 10.1 *(continued)*

Year(s)	*Author(s)*	*Substance*	*Dosage and route of administration*	*Indication*	*Effect*	*Side-effects*
(VI) Vitamins: Mechanism(s) of action – stabilization of lysosomal membranes, cofactor for hydroxydehydrogenase (estradiol synthesis)						
1977	Lithgow and Politzer	Vitamin A	2 × 25 000 IU/day; oral for 15 days	Menorrhagia	+	None
(VII) Animal peptide organ extract: Mechanism(s) of action – estrogen hyperactivity, antagonism of vasopressin, bradykinin, histamine, and carbachol						
1976	Rendina and Patrono	'Lysometra' (low MW polypeptides	2.5 ml i.m.; days 5–25, three cycles maximum	Menorrhagia	+	None
(VIII) Vasopressin derivatives: Mechanism(s) of action – vasoconstriction and uterine contraction						
	Tauber and Nohlen[b]	t-GLVP (Triglycyl-vasopressin)	2 ml of 0.1 mg/ml i.v.; day 2	IUD patients	+	Facial paleness
(IX) Chemical cytotoxic agents: Mechanism of action – chemical curettage of endometrial cavity						
1969	Zipper *et al.*	Ethanol 100% or ethanol–2% formalin	2 ml intrauterine immediately after menstrual period	IUD patients	+	Sterility
(X) Benzamide derivatives: Mechanism(s) of action – effect on hypothalamic–hypophyseal axis (gonadotrophin release), decreases ovarian sensitivity to gonadotrophins, endometrial hypertrophy						
1977	Trévoux	Sulpiridin	3 × 50 mg/day; oral for 6 weeks	IUD patients and menorrhagia patients	+	Weight gain, amenorrhea, galactorrhea

[a] KIU = Kallikrein inactivator units
[b] Unpublished observations

optimizing their adaptation in the uterine cavity have been developed, a more promising approach may be in the use of drugs capable of interfering with the uterine bleeding mechanism(s). A wide variety of such substances has been used clinically with variable success (Table 10.1). Among these drugs, proteinase inhibitors deserve particular attention.

PATHOPHYSIOLOGICAL CONSIDERATIONS

Excessive uterine bleeding may present itself in well-defined clinical conditions such as increased or prolonged menstrual bleeding (hypermenorrhea/menorrhagia), intermenstrual bleeding (spotting), or a combination of both types of hemorrhage. This may or may not be accompanied by spastic cramps in the lower abdomen or back (dysmenorrhea). The amount of excess blood loss is usually dependent upon the type of IUD which is used. The pathophysiological mechanisms which cause uterine hemorrhage have not yet been fully elucidated, neither in normal menstruation nor in atypical, excessive uterine bleeding during the course of intrauterine contraception. A number of detailed investigations indicate that the bleeding etiology is multifactorial, including morphological changes of the endometrium and several biochemical mediator systems such as the blood coagulation–fibrinolysis system, the kallikrein–kinin system and the complement system. The desired contraceptive effect of the IUD and the occurrence of excessive uterine bleeding or other side-effects probably arise from a common basis.

Morphological aspects

Morphologically, one might suspect that the obvious explanation for the cause of excess hemorrhage experienced with IUD use would be the development of mechanical erosions in the soft endometrial tissue which lead to the exposure and/or traumatization of superficial endometrial vessels. However, direct mechanical surface damage of the endometrium does not appear to be of major importance (Hohman *et al.,* 1977), since most of the endometria of IUD-wearing women are intact as found by gross as well as microscopic examination, despite surface degeneration and denudation of variable degrees. Moreover, the superficial or even deeper erosions and/or ulcerations are not sufficient in number to explain the excess amount of bleeding during menstrual periods (Hohman *et al.,* 1977; Ludwig *et al.,* 1976; Moyer *et al.,* 1978). Additionally, no correlation exists between the histological findings and excessive hemorrhage with or without the IUD (Morse *et al.,* 1966; Moyer and Mishell, 1971).

Vessel defects which do not represent a completely open lumen, but rather gaps, can be found in increased quantities in the area of the endometrium in contact with the IUD. Such gaps may be explained through the occurrence of shear forces which are provoked by the device in a pressurized, atrophic or necrotic endometrium (Hohman *et al.,* 1977). These shear forces may lead to torsion or to a forced stretching of the vessels, and may also cause degeneration of endothelial cells as a consequence of IUD pressure upon the superficial endometrium. Since all degrees of such degeneration are present in the endometrium when an IUD is in place it can be assumed that vessel damage is not a one-time occurrence, but rather is a morphological result of a continuously acting noxa throughout the cycle (Ancla *et al.,* 1967; Hohman *et al.,* 1977). The extravasation of red blood cells and plasma through the above-mentioned gaps during any time in the menstrual cycle therefore offers a morphologically based explanation at least for the etiology of intermenstrual spotting (Hohman *et al.,* 1977; Rybo, 1978), but does not satisfactorily explain increased or prolonged menstrual bleeding.

This might also be the reason for the clinical observation that treatment of IUD-associated uterine hemorrhage with exogenous estrogens is usually not successful. The proliferative stimulus of estrogen necessary for cessation of bleeding cannot reach the endometrium that is under pressure (i.e. under the IUD). Other morphological changes observed in endometria with IUDs may also indicate the influence of biochemical factors in the uterine environment. Among these are interstitial edema with extravasation of red blood cells and the nearly complete lack of local blood coagulation (Moyer and Mishell, 1971; Moyer *et al.,* 1978), and also increased vessel permeability and capillary fragility. The reduction of bleeding by combined treatment with vitamin C and iron (Hefnawi and Yacout, 1978), or other drugs known to increase capillary resistance, provides evidence for the correct interpretation of these morphological findings.

A third morphological phenomenon which may explain excess bleeding occurring after longer IUD use – i.e. more than 6 months – is the observation of endometrial polyposis, as shown in Figure 10.1. Such endometrial polyps are found in most endometrial specimens, particularly when copper-containing IUDs have been in place longer than 6 months, as can be demonstrated with the combination of histology and scanning electronmicroscopy (Ludwig, 1980). Movements of the IUD may disrupt or tear off the polyps, causing surface epithelial defects which may contribute substantially to uterine hemorrhage.

Biochemical aspects

Despite the biochemical consequences of endometrial-cell necrosis, the main influence in the intrauterine environment after insertion of an IUD is exerted by leukocytic elements. Shortly after insertion, large numbers of inflammatory cells migrate into the uterine cavity, particularly polymorphonuclear granulocytes and macrophages (Moyer and Shaw, 1973). The uterus becomes the arena of a foreign-body reaction, the suggested cascade mechanism of which is shown in Figure 10.2. Generally, the situation is similar to that observed during regenerative inflammation, also called 'sterile inflammation', the latter under the assumption that pathogenic bacteria are absent. However, this is not always the case, since pathogenic bacteria have been found on many IUDs (Feichter *et al.,* 1978). The destruction of cellular elements in the uterine cavity and alterations of the intrauterine environment caused by the regenerative inflammatory process leads to the liberation of highly active proteolytic enzymes and to the activation of various humoral mediator systems.

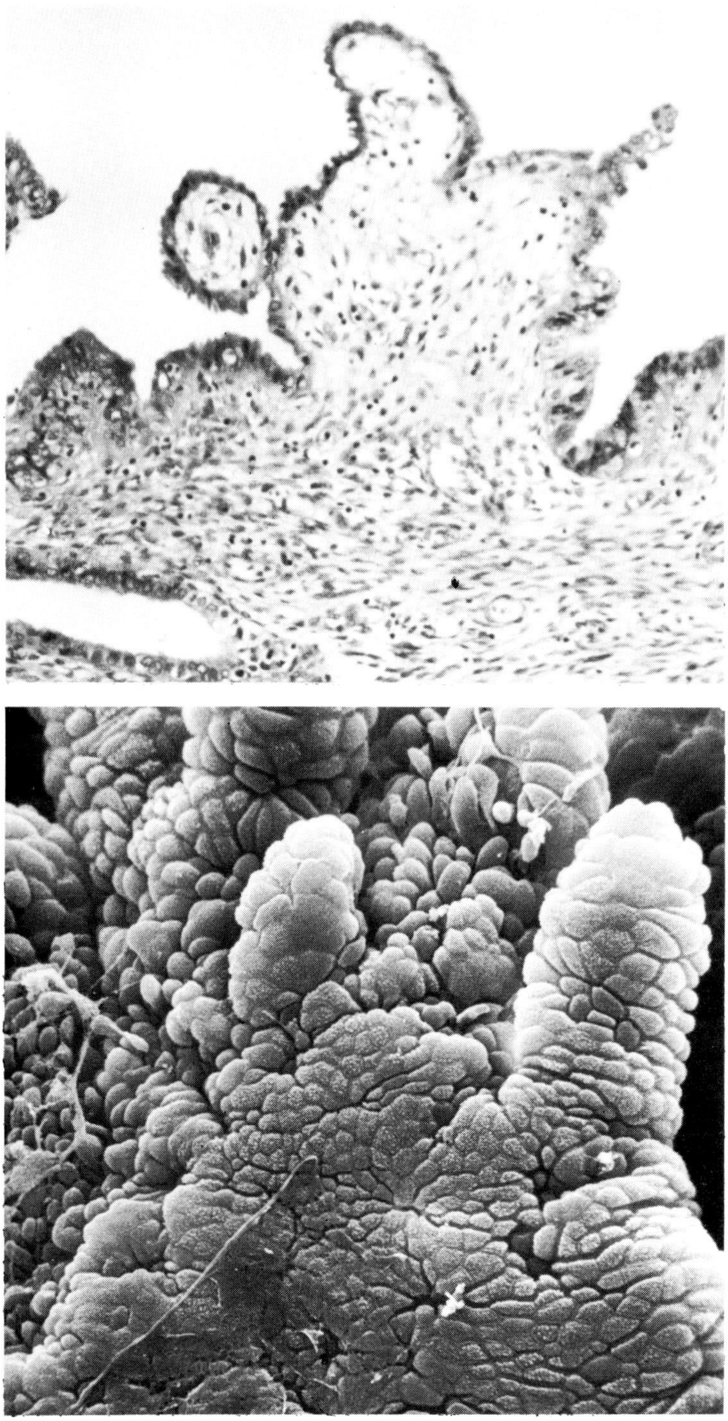

Figure 10.1 Demonstration of endometrial polyps developed in response to the presence of an IUD. Tearing of these polyps by IUD friction may lead to surface defects which contribute to excess uterine bleeding. The polyps represent a more or less consistent finding, particularly in endometria with copper IUDs in place for longer than 6 months.(a) Scanning electronmicrograph demonstrating endometrial surface in contact with a copper-containing IUD, in place for 20 months. Tissue was obtained after hysterectomy on the 19th day of the cycle (early secretory phase). A multitude of endometrial polyps are present, varying in size; polypoidal surface cells appear flattened and polygonal in shape, and the cell borders are clearly visible. Magnification × 500. (b) Corresponding histological section of an endometrial area adjacent to the tissue subjected to scanning electronmicroscopy. Mild, transient endometritis is present, as indicated by the occasional presence of white blood cells spread throughout the subepithelial stroma. Magnification × 150; haematoxylin and eosin staining

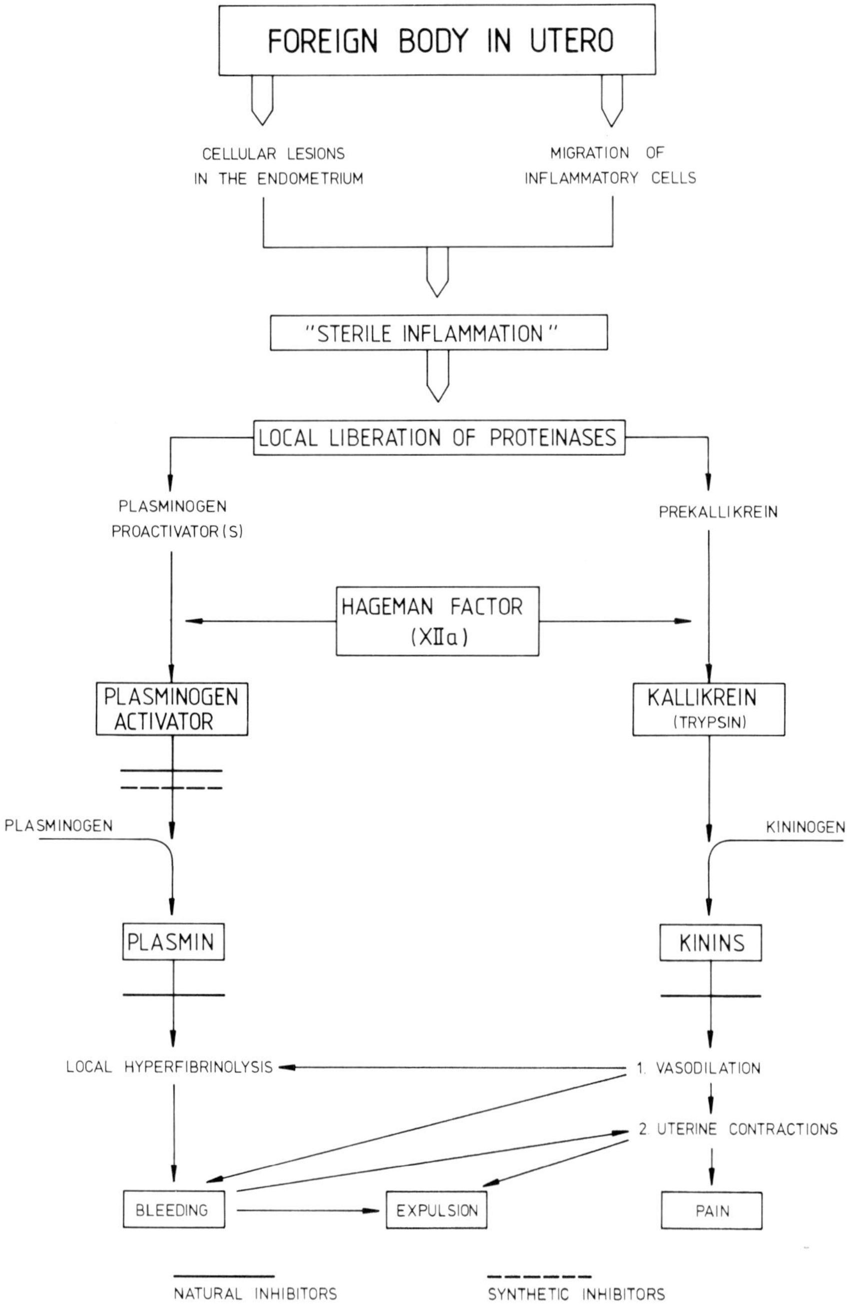

Figure 10.2 Suggested biochemical cascade for mechanism of development of IUD side-effects including bleeding, expulsion, and pain. Main enzymes used are plasmin and kinins. Points of inhibition with natural and/or synthetic proteinase inhibitors are indicated

Activation of the fibrinolysis system and the kallikrein–kinin system are particularly important since they result in the generation of plasmin and kinins. Local generation of plasmin is equivalent to local hyperfibrinolysis, which in turn interferes with local blood clotting. In contrast, liberated kinins exert pharmacological effects that may also explain the symptoms seen in the bleeding IUD patient. Under inflammatory conditions, kinins cause vasodilation and increased vascular permeability; they also act upon smooth muscle to affect contraction, and cause pain when they come in contact with free nerve endings. These pharmacological events also explain other IUD-associated complications such as expulsion and/or dysmenorrheic complaints. Prostaglandins have not been included in this cascade mechanism, but their influence on the development of IUD-associated uterine hemorrhage and of other IUD side-effects has been postulated (Saksena and Harper, 1974; Barry, 1975). The effective reduction of IUD-induced uterine bleeding through the oral administration of prostaglandin synthetase inhibitors presents at least partial evidence of a causal relationship between prostaglandins and the etiology of this bleeding (Damarawy and Toppozada, 1976; Guillebaud *et al.,* 1978).

Human endometrium contains large amounts of fibrinolysis activator(s). Their local concentration is dependent upon the stage of the menstrual cycle, reaching the highest values shortly before the onset of menstruation (Rybo, 1966). The greatest concentration of plasminogen activator(s) is found at endometrial areas close to the fundus of the uterus (Tauber, 1979a). This may at least partially explain the higher amount of blood loss experienced with IUDs whose vertical arm is located in this area, such as the Lippes Loop. High fibrinolytic activity may also account for the lack of coagulability of menstrual blood (Nilsson, 1975). Women suffering from menorrhagia exhibit high fibrinolytic activity in their menstrual blood (Rybo, 1966). Plasminogen activators are a part of the enzymatic makeup of leukocytes (Unkeless *et al.,* 1974), as are other proteolytic enzymes such as collagenase and elastase. Increased fibrinolysis (proteolysis) potential can also be demonstrated in the endometrial tissue of IUD-wearing women (Larsson *et al.,* 1974; Bonnar *et al.,* 1976), although the higher plasminogen activator activity is not always reflected in endometrial secretions when an IUD is in place (Tauber, 1979a). This is most likely due to the local presence of inhibitors of fibrinolysis which control proteolytic processes in the body. One of the functions of the inhibitors is also to protect epithelial surfaces from proteolysis. However, when high concentrations of proteolytic activity are present, much or all of the inhibitor may be bound to enzyme, causing a local deficiency of inhibitory activity (Krumme *et al.,* 1977). The endometrium and the uterine secretions of IUD-wearing women suffering from hypermenorrhea show a lack of α_1-antitrypsin activity (Tauber *et al.,* 1977a), which is known to be an inhibitor of both plasmin and kallikrein and is also capable of inhibiting proteinases of leukocytic origin such as elastase and collagenase.

From the above-presented considerations it may be concluded that the main pathophysiological moment in IUD generation of uterine hemorrhage is the impairment of local mechanisms of hemostasis, which is maintained by the presence of the device. This impairment is caused by: (1) a local hyperfibrinolysis, e.g. proteolysis of varying degrees; and (2) a local decrease in physiological inhibitory activity, at least temporarily, while the IUD is in place.

Irrespective of other mechanisms which may also be included in the etiology of IUD-associated bleeding, it must be the goal of treatment to reduce or eliminate the hemostatic impairment, i.e. to either suppress the hyperfibrinolytic reaction or offer suitable inhibitors for compensation of their local deficiency. The combination of both therapeutic principles can be found when synthetic and/or natural inhibitors of fibrinolysis are applied.

TREATMENT WITH PROTEINASE INHIBITORS

Synthetic proteinase inhibitors

The most commonly used synthetic inhibitors are epsilon aminocaproic acid (EACA; 6-aminohexanoic acid) and its cyclic derivative, tranexamic acid (AMCA; *trans*-4-(aminomethyl)-cyclohexane carbonic acid). Due to their clinical importance and common use, the pharmacological effects of both substances are relatively well known from *in vitro* and *in vivo* studies (Iwamoto, 1975; Nilsson, 1975). EACA and AMCA have low molecular weights and are inhibitors particularly of the plasminogen activation induced by tissue activators. Inhibition results from the generation of irreversible plasminogen–inhibitor complexes in a ratio of 1:1 for EACA and 1:2 for AMCA. Formation of these complexes is accompanied by a structural change in the plasminogen molecule, which then loses its ability for activation to plasmin (Iwamoto, 1975). Concentrations higher than 10^{-4} mol/l AMCA also inhibit plasmin, the end-products of plasminogen activation, by binding to the plasmin molecule and thereby decreasing its fibrin-directed lytic activity. Owing to its longer retention in tissues, AMCA exhibits an inhibitory capacity 5–8 fold higher than EACA. The simultaneous presence of natural antiplasmins (plasma proteinase inhibitors) enforces this inhibitory capacity. EACA and AMCA may be administered orally, intravenously, intramuscularly, and locally. Synthetic antifibrinolytics are excreted mainly via the kidney, and are therefore strongly contraindicated in patients with chronic renal disease.

The toxicity of these substances is low (Melander *et al.,* 1965), although side-effects such as diarrhea, abdominal pain, nausea, headache, dizziness, and orthostatic complaints have been observed even at therapeutic doses (Ludwig and Mehring, 1965; Weström and Bengtsson, 1970; Nilsson and Rybo, 1971; see Table 10.1). These are less pronounced for AMCA than EACA and do not occur when either of the inhibitors is applied locally. EACA should not be administered systemically during pregnancy since animal studies have shown retardation of embryological development (Melander *et al.,* 1965), although the local application of small amounts of EACA (released from intrauterine devices) has not confirmed these observations (Andrade *et al.,* 1978).

Reduction of bleeding by oral administration of EACA and/or AMCA in

IUD-associated uterine hemorrhage has been proved (Weström and Bengtsson, 1970; Kasonde and Bonnar, 1975; see Table 10.1). Disadvantages of the oral administration of these drugs are the large amounts required for effective treatment, the resulting side-effects, the short duration of effectiveness, and therefore the necessity to repeat the treatment with every menstrual period.

Natural proteinase inhibitors

The only natural inhibitor used therapeutically to date is aprotinin, a basic polypeptide containing 58 amino acids with a molecular weight of approximately 6000 daltons. Aprotinin originates from bovine organs and inhibits numerous estero-proteolytic enzymes such as kallikreins, acrosin, trypsin, plasmin, chymotrypsin, and proteinases from leukocytes or damaged tissue. Since aprotinin is a true antifibrinolytic, it inhibits the plasmin–fibrin reaction as well as plasminogen activation by the proactivator(s). Accordingly, aprotinin works by inhibiting and regulating mechanisms of the fibrinolysis and coagulation systems, the kallikrein–kinin system, and the complement system. When compared with synthetic inhibitors, aprotinin possesses the largest inhibitory capacity against the above-mentioned enzymes (Umezawa, 1972).

The chemistry, pharmacokinetics, and pharmacology of aprotinin are well known and defined in clinical use. This inhibitor can be administered intravenously and/or locally. As a peptide it is of no value when given orally. Local application of aprotinin has been successful in the treatment of various inflammatory diseases such as arthritis and non-specific vaginitis. The inflammatory reaction at the endometrial surface epithelium in the presence of an IUD can also be effectively reduced through local application of aprotinin (Tauber *et al.,* 1978).

LOCAL INTRAUTERINE APPLICATION OF PROTEINASE INHIBITORS IN INTRAUTERINE CONTRACEPTION

In order to circumvent the disadvantages of systemic application of proteinase inhibitors used against IUD-induced hypermenorrhea and/or menorrhagia, local intrauterine application of these agents is indicated. In general, there are two modes of such application: (1) the instillation of an inhibitor solution into the uterine cavity; and (2) the release of inhibitors from depots which are bound to the IUD and exert their local effect over a long period of time ('medicated devices').

If one considers the presence of a delicate hemostatic balance between the blood coagulation and fibrinolysis systems in peripheral circulation the question arises as to whether inhibitors might be absorbed from local application sites (i.e. intrauterine) to such a degree that thrombophilic predisposition would develop. This would of course narrow the therapeutic usefulness of the intrauterine application of inhibitors. To answer this question, gelatin capsules containing various amounts of proteinase inhibitors were put into the uterine cavities of women 3 days after dilation and curettage, the latter being a treatment which should allow for almost complete absorption. Blood was collected by venipuncture at various times before and after insertion of capsules, which dissolve between 30 and 60 minutes after contact with uterine fluid. Plasminogen-activator activity in peripheral plasma was measured by radial enzyme diffusion (Schumacher and Schill, 1972) and the results expressed in human urokinase equivalents. No major inhibition of plasminogen activation was found up to 6 hours after administration of pharmacological doses (up to 100 mg EACA and AMCA, or up to 100 000 KIU (kallikrein inactivator units) or aprotinin; Table 10.2). This shows that not large enough quantities of the drugs were absorbed, even in these most susceptible uteri, to interfere with the peripheral fibrinolysis system.

Table 10.2 Inhibition of plasminogen activation in peripheral plasma after intrauterine application of antifibrinolytic agents[a]

	Time of blood withdrawal (min):												
	EACA				*AMCA*				*Aprotinin*[b]				
Dosage (mg)	0	30	180	360	0	30	180	360	0	10	20	30	60
10	110	102	125	117	128	135	125	142	128	112	132	135	142
50	117	114	116	110									
100	114	142	87	134	95	82	73	106	135	108	150	145	145
500	100	135	71	35	157	142	128	65					

[a] Substrate, bovine fibrinogen (Behring Diagnostics); standard, human urokinase, 2160 U/ml (M.R.C. reference preparation); method of determination, radial enzyme diffusion (Schumacher and Schill, 1972); form of application, sterile gelatin capsules into uterine cavity; time of application, 3 days after dilatation and curettage. Each value represents mean from three patients. Values are given in human urokinase equivalents

[b] Aprotinin was given in doses of 10000 and 100000 KIU (upper and lower lines, respectively), both dosages containing approximately 0.3 μg protein

Instillation of inhibitor solutions into the uterine cavity

Local administration of inhibitor solutions is indicated in cases of hypermenorrhea, menorrhagia and/or spotting which are caused by the presence of an IUD. Before treatment, any inflammatory diseases of the fallopian tubes and/or ovaries should be excluded by bimanual pelvic examination, and the common parameters which are indicative of inflammation such as blood sedimentation rate, WBC count, differential cell count, and body temperature should be evaluated. It is very important that all diagnostic measures be performed in cases in which the presence of a genital malignoma, ectopic pregnancy or miscarriage are suspected, all of which are known to produce abnormal uterine bleeding. In these cases, local treatment with proteinase inhibitors is contraindicated.

The use of stronger inhibiting substances (those with higher inhibitory capacity, such as AMCA and aprotinin) should be considered preferentially. In patients with dysmenorrhea, the application of aprotinin is recommended since it also relieves pain through inhibition of kinin liberation. Commercially available aprotinin solutions (i.e. between 10000 and 20000 KIU/ml) are satisfactory for successful treatment.

The application of inhibitor solutions can be performed either at the occasion of IUD insertion in patients who are expected to develop heavy bleeding, or perimenstrually daily or every second day when menorrhagia is present. Spotting should be treated at any time it occurs, particularly when the patient comes to the office with complaints. Treatment can be repeated over several consecutive days, although in our experience not more than three applications are required to stop the hemorrhage.

For intrauterine administration of inhibitor solutions, the vaginal portion of the uterus is exposed by inserting a speculum into the vagina, and the area is disinfected. The cervix should be fixed with a tenaculum, although this can sometimes be omitted. The commercially available sterile inhibitor solution is drawn into a disposable tuberculin syringe equipped with a slightly bent steel cannula having a smooth tip. The cannula is carefully inserted into the cervical canal, up to the uterine fundus (Figure 10.3). The solution is administered slowly to prevent reflux from the cervical canal as well as patient discomfort. The use of a steel cannula as compared with a plastic catheter offers the advantage that it also allows for sounding of the uterus and, particularly, correct intrauterine placement of the IUD. The volume applied into the uterine cavity is approximately 1–2 ml. Our experience with local treatment of uterine cavity for the reduction of IUD-associated bleeding showed that menorrhagia caused by various types of devices could be reduced from an average of 8.5 days to 4.5 days duration, i.e. by approximately 50%. For decrease of bleeding, both AMCA and aprotinin were equally effective (Tauber *et al.*, 1977b).

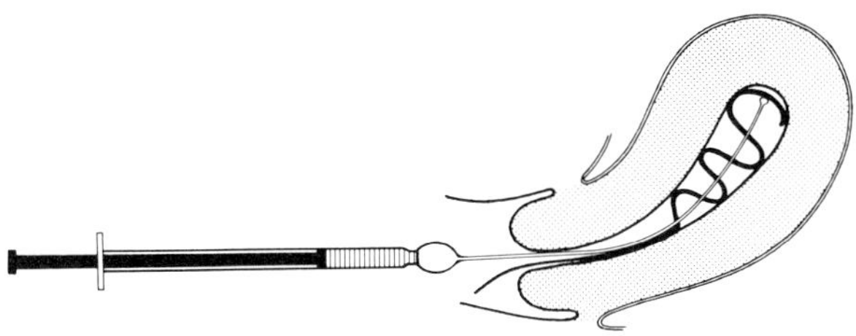

Figure 10.3 Schematic illustration of the intrauterine application of inhibitor solutions in IUD-wearing patients. The inhibitor is injected with a disposable tuberculin syringe fitted with a steel cannula having a smooth tip, which is inserted up to the uterine fundus (from Tauber, 1976)

When physiological saline was similarly administered as a control, no influence on bleeding was observed, or the intensity and duration of the hemorrhage increased. This was the case even in patients who were treated successfully with inhibitor solutions. The duration of success (decrease of bleeding) in most patients lasted for at least three cycles. In some cases, bleeding could be completely normalized.

If the treatment with proteinase inhibitors remains unsuccessful, other causes should be considered such as displacement of IUD, including partial or complete perforation of the myometrial walls or cervical localization of the device. In such cases removal of the IUD is mandatory. Although the local application of proteinase inhibitors in IUD-associated hemorrhage is a rather complicated venture since it requires manipulation by the physician under sterile conditions, the fact that only low amounts of inhibitor have to be administered for success is advantageous. In addition, the cessation of bleeding allows for continuation of the IUD as a contraceptive.

Treatment of uterine hemorrhage with antifibrinolytically active intrauterine devices (medicated IUDs)

The efforts to successfully reduce IUD-associated uterine hemorrhage by local application of proteinase inhibitor solutions have led to the development of intrauterine devices which carry such substances to obtain a long-lasting effect by steady diffusion of inhibitor into the uterine environment. The major problem encountered with this approach is the development of an adequate matrix which will allow for a continuous release of the inhibitor in sufficient quantities. The molecular weight of inhibitors and therefore their ability to diffuse from the matrix has also to be considered. The first animal experiments with EACA–Silicone tubes linked to IUDs were encouraging (Shaw *et al.,* 1975; Andrade *et al.,* 1978); uterine hemorrhage could be reduced to only one-third of the original amount of bleeding. Studies in women also showed hemorrhage-reducing effects even when different types of intrauterine devices and different inhibitors were used (Ragab and Thomas, 1976; Hefnawi *et al.,* 1977).

A randomized study was performed at our institution to investigate the effects on uterine hemorrhage of local EACA release from silicone tubes containing this proteinase inhibitor (Tauber *et al.,* 1979). Women were fitted with intrauterine devices and menstrual blood loss (MBL) was determined from the tampons and napkins collected during menstruation. Three types of IUDs were used: commercially available Multiload copper IUDs exposing a copper surface area of 250 mm^2 to the uterine environment (ML Cu-250); Multiload devices without copper wire, i.e. plain devices which were equal in shape and material but with a silicone tube pushed over the vertical arm (ML Silastic, see Figure 10.4); and plain Multiload IUDs which carried a similar silicone tube containing 24 mg of the proteinase inhibitor EACA (ML EACA). The *in vitro* release rate of EACA from the silicone tube had been determined previously as being approximately 50 ug/day (International Fertility Research Program, Research Triangle Park, N.C., USA). The Multiload IUD skeleton was used because of its superior performance in our clinic with respect to almost all IUD-associated events. Each group of patients consisted of approximately 35 women (range 33–37). MBL was calculated after determining the iron content (measured by atomic absorption analysis) of the menstrual blood eluted from the tampon and napkin material which had been collected during the last menstrual period before IUD insertion, and during the first, second, third, and sixth postinsertion menstrual periods.

All groups of patients exhibited increased menstrual blood loss after insertion of devices. In the group of patients receiving EACA-medicated IUDs, however, a pronounced and statistically significant ($p<0.05$)

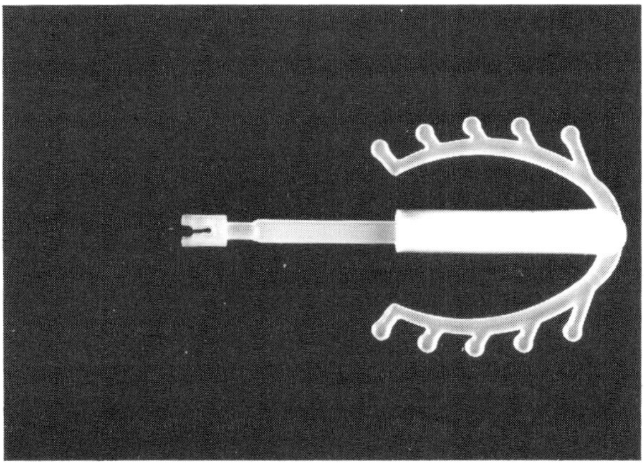

Figure 10.4 Plain Multiload IUD skeleton with a silicone-EACA tube fitted onto the vertical arm (ML–EACA) (from Tauber, 1979b)

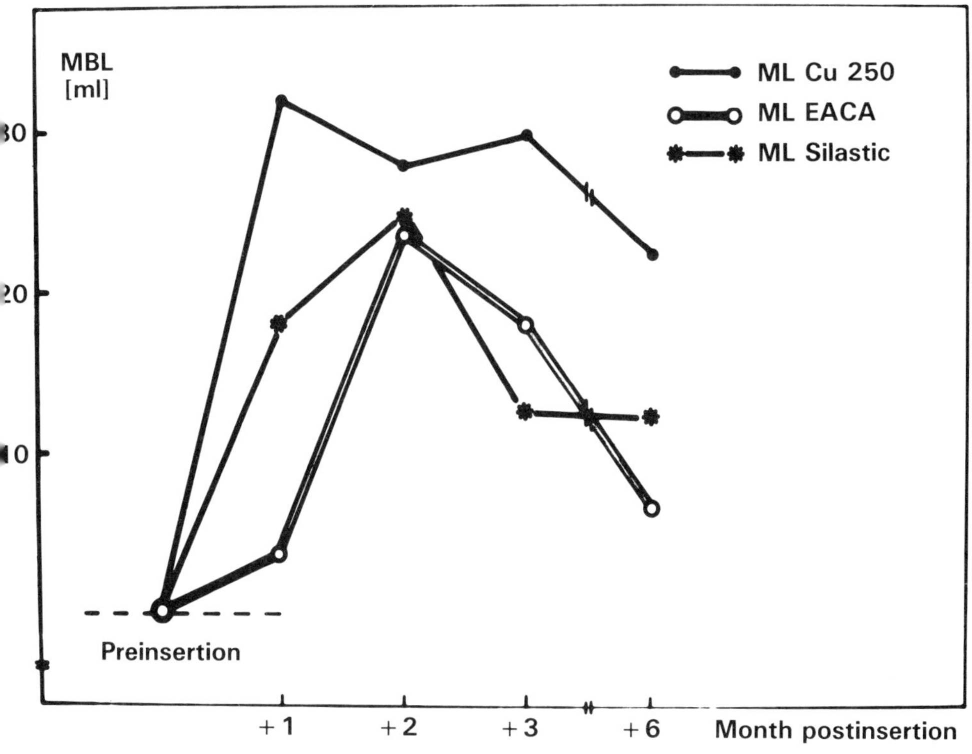

Figure 10.5 Mean menstrual blood loss (MBL) of women fitted with various ML IUDs. MBL was determined the month before insertion (preinsertion) and 1, 2, 3, and 6 months postinsertion. The data presented have been normalized because of the large variability of preinsertion MBL between subjects. Note general increase of MBL in all groups after insertion with the exception of the first month postinsertion for ML–EACA users (from Tauber, (1979b)

reduction of the average menstrual blood loss during the first menstrual period after insertion was noted as compared with the group of women receiving ML Cu-250 IUDs (Figure 10.5).

In the following cycles the blood loss among the different groups was almost equal and decreased to the lowest values in the sixth month after insertion. Obviously, the antifibrinolytic agent released locally from the IUD can reduce blood loss at least for the first menstrual period after insertion, although the effect is not maintained during further cycles when this particular device is used. This emphasizes the usefulness of this type of therapy, but also reveals that the inhibitor-releasing matrix is certainly not ideal as yet. The short-term effectiveness of this releasing system could be due to either a release rate of EACA from the matrix that is too fast, and/or the fact that the amount of inhibitor on each IUD is too small. Other techniques for inhibitor linkage to IUDs such as microencapsulation and/or the use of biodegradable carrier matrices may allow for the application of larger amounts of inhibitor. Future efforts should therefore be aimed at developing better inhibitor-releasing systems for the successful reduction of IUD-associated uterine hemorrhage.

CONCLUDING REMARKS

Uterine bleeding remains the most prominent and widespread problem associated with the use of contraceptive intrauterine devices. Various hypotheses have been developed to account for all the pathophysiological aspects of the hemorrhage and, based upon these, a variety of treatment regimens have been suggested. Some of these regimens have been successful, though not in all women, and others have failed. Treatment should be individualized, and its success depends on correct physiological understanding and therefore on the drugs used.

In most instances of IUD-associated hemorrhage, both morphological and biochemical alterations in the uterine environment offer combined grounds for this pathological condition. Morphologically, three aspects of endometrial changes appear relevant: (1) the occurrence of flat erosions in the endometrial layer, although these cannot sufficiently explain heavy bleeding; (2) the presence of gaps in the endometrial vessels which are caused by IUD pressure; and (3) the observation of endometrial polyps varying in size which arise from small endometrial bases and are easily torn off by IUD movements. This would leave the epithelium with numerous defects which may contribute to the bleeding. While erosions and, particularly, gaps represent consistent findings in IUD-affected endometria over all periods of IUD use, polyps occur mainly in women wearing copper IUDs for over 6 months. This may account for the 'late bleeders', i.e. those who bleed after a longer interval without hemorrhage after insertion.

The most obvious biochemical explanation for the occurrence of bleeding appears to be the intrauterine activation of various humoral enzyme systems, such as the local fibrinolysis system and the kinin system, by the presence of the IUD. The overall result is the impairment of mechanisms which are responsible for local hemostasis, and consequently bleeding

Table 10.3 Effects of proteinase inhibitors on mammalian reproductive processes in the female genital tract

Reference	*Event investigated*	*Test system used*	*Inhibitor used*	*Results*
Zaneveld *et al.* (1971)	Fertilization *in vivo*	Capacitation test with rabbit gametes	Pancreatic trypsin inhibitor	91% inhibition of fertilization
Schumacher and Zaneveld (1974)	Spermatozoa – cervical mucus penetration *in vitro*	Slide test with human gametes	Aprotinin	Significant reduction in number of penetrating spermatozoa
Yang *et al.* (1976)	Fertilization *in vivo*	Capacitation test with rabbit gametes	Aprotinin	5[a] – no significant effect; 50[a] – 60% decrease of fertilization; 100[a] – 90% decrease of fertilization
Denker (1976)	Blastolemmase activity *in vitro* and *in vivo*	Gelatin substrate film test and rabbit blastocyst	Aprotinin and EACA	Aprotinin: complete inhibition (long lasting) EACA: no effect/no inhibition
Tauber and Wolf (1975); Wolf *et al.* (1975); Tauber *et al.* (1977b)	IUD-induced uterine bleeding	Intrauterine administration to women	Aprotinin (up to three 1 ml injections of 19 mg/ml each day for 3 days maximum)	Significant decrease of bleeding; no pregnancies
Andrade *et al.* (1978)	Fertilization and implantation *in vivo*	Oral and intrauterine (impregnated IUDs) administration to rabbits	EACA (oral, 375 mg kg^{-1} day^{-1} in four doses; intrauterine 4 mg)	Both oral and intrauterine administration had no effect on fertilization or implantation rates compared with controls
Tauber *et al.* (unpublished observations)	IUD-induced uterine bleeding	Intrauterine administration (impregnated IUDs) to women	EACA, 24 mg	Significant decrease of bleeding; no pregnancies

[a] Results given in $\mu g/5 \times 10^4$ spermatozoa in 0.5 ml

occurs. Indirect evidence for this biochemical concept is provided by successful use of various proteinase inhibitors (known as antifibrinolytic agents, and including EACA, AMCA, and aprotinin) when they are applied locally through either intrauterine instillation or release from an IUD.

With respect to the above, attention should be drawn to a second important aspect of practical relevance in the treatment of IUD-associated uterine hemorrhage with proteinase inhibitors. These inhibitors not only influence the pathophysiology of bleeding, but also interact with reproductive processes which occur at the tubal and/or uterine level (Table 10.3). A number of animal investigations indicate that, among the inhibitors, at least aprotinin can effectively reduce or even prevent the fertilizing capacity of spermatozoa *in vivo* (Zaneveld *et al.,* 1971), and that this drug is also effective in blocking the dissolution of the blastocyst coverings and implantation initiation by the inhibition of an enzyme (blastolemmase) which appears to be important for these processes in the rabbit uterus (Denker, 1976). The presence of aprotinin in the uterine cavity, either released by an IUD or injected through the cervical canal, would therefore add to the contraceptive effect of the device while simultaneously minimizing the occurrence of uterine hemorrhage.

A further indication for such an influence is that in our patients, after aprotinin instillation into the uteri of IUD wearers, no pregnancies were encountered, although initially expected. This is rather surprising if one considers the initial assumption that the contraceptive effect of the IUD may derive from the same pathophysiological basis as do side-effects (such as bleeding). The decrease of side-effects by proteinase inhibitor treatment should, if the assumption is correct, lead to partial or even complete loss of IUD contraceptive effectiveness. From these observations it appears most likely that the two processes, interference with fertilization and implantation through the presence of the IUD and occurrence of side-effects, affect different proteinases. More specifically, it is likely that the inhibition of plasminogen activation or plasmin has no effect on the IUD-induced prevention of blastocyst implantation and/or development.

Only Lippes Loops with attached *aprotinin*-containing matrices, made from biodegradable collagen, have been developed to the stage of clinical investigation. Results are discouraging, however, since the problems arising with these IUDs have been similar to those experienced with the Multiload-EACA devices, i.e. long-term release is not obtained for technical reasons. Future research in this field should therefore be aimed at the development of IUDs with proteinase inhibitors and releasing systems that allow for slow biodegeneration of the matrix in the uterus.

Acknowledgments

A portion of this work was supported by PARFR Grant 81 N. We are grateful to Dr A. Klöppel for performing the atomic absorption analyses to determine menstrual blood loss.

References

Ancla, M., de Brux, J. and Simon, P. (1967). Aneurysmal microthrombosis associated with intrauterine devices in the human endometrium. *Lab. Invest.*, **17**, 61

Anderson, A. B. M., Guillebaud, J., Haynes, P. J. and Turnbull, A. C. (1976). Reduction of menstrual blood-loss by prostaglandin-synthetase inhibitors. *Lancet*, **1**, 774

Andrade, A. T. L., Shaw, S. T., Jr. and Guerra, M. O. (1978). Effects of epsilon-amino-caproic acid on fertility in the rabbit. *J. Reprod. Fertil.*, **52**, 261

Barry, M. A. (1975). PG's synthesis by cell population adherent to IUCD. Presented at the *International Conference on Prostaglandins*, Florence, May

Bonnar, J., Kasonde, J. M., Haddon, M. and Hassanein, K. (1976). Fibrinolytic activity *in utero* and bleeding complications with intrauterine contraceptive devices. *Br. J. Obstet. Gynaecol.*, **83**, 160

Callender, S. T., Warner, G. T. and Cope, E. (1970). Treatment of menorrhagia with tranexamic acid. A double blind trial. *Br. Med. J.*, **4**, 214

Damarawy, H. and Toppozada, M. (1976). Control of bleeding due to IUDs by prostaglandin biosynthesis inhibitor. *IRCS Med. Sci.*, **4**, 5

Denker, H.-W. (1976). Interaction of proteinase inhibitors with blastocyst proteinases involved in implantation. In Peeters, H. (ed.) *Protides of the Biological Fluids*, 23rd Colloquium, p. 63. (Oxford: Pergamon Press)

Feichter, G. E., Tauber, P. F., Rosenthal, E. and Ludwig, H. (1978). Zur bakteriellen Besiedelung kupferhaltiger Intrauterinpessare. *Geburtsh. Frauenheilk.*, **38**, 904

Genicot, R. (1978). Le traitement des saignements dus aux stérilets par un inhibiteur de protéinases. *Rev. Med. Liege*, **33**, 183

Guillebaud, J., Anderson, A. B. M. and Turnbull, A. C. (1978). Reduction by mefenamic acid of increased menstrual blood loss associated with intrauterine contraception. *Br. J. Obstet. Gynaecol.*, **85**, 53

Harrison, R. F. and Campbell, S. (1976). A double-blind trial of ethamsylate in the treatment of primary and intrauterine-device hemorrhage. *Lancet*, **2**, 283

Hefnawi, F. and Yacout, M. M. (1978). Intrauterine contraception in developing countries. In Ludwig, H. and Tauber, P. F. (eds.) *Human Fertilization*, p. 249. (Stuttgart: Thieme Verlag)

Hefnawi, F., Yacout, M. M., Hosni, M., El-Sheika, Z. and Hassanein, M. (1977). Medicated intrauterine devices to improve bleeding events. *Int. J. Gynaecol. Obstet.*, **15**, 79

Hohman, W. R., Shaw, S. T., Jr., Macanlay, L. and Moyer, D. L. (1977). Vascular defects in human endometrium caused by intrauterine contraceptive devices. *Contraception*, **16**, 507

Iwamoto, M. (1975). Plasminogen-plasmin system. IX. Specific binding of tranexamic acid to plasmin. *Thrombos. Diathes. Haemorrh. (Stuttg.)*, **33**, 573

Kasonde, J. M. and Bonnar, J. (1975). Aminocaproic acid and menstrual blood loss in women using intrauterine devices. *Br. Med. J.*, **302**, 17

Kovács, L. and Annus, J. (1978). Wirksamkeit von Etamsylat bei der durch Intrauterin-pessare ausgelösten Menorrhagie. *Gynecol. Obstet. Invest.*, **9**, 161

Krumme, D., Wallner, O. and Fritz, H. (1977). Proteinases and proteinase inhibitors in human cervical mucus - selected properties in view of their clinical relevance. In Insler, U. and Bettendorf, G. (eds.) *The Uterine Cervix In Reproduction*, p. 92. (Stuttgart: Thieme Verlag)

Larsson, B., Liedholm, P., Sjöberg, N. O. and Astedt, B. (1974). Increased fibrinolytic activity in the endometrium of patients using copper-IUD. *Contraception*, **9**, 531

Lauder, M. M. and Lauder, A. D. (1977). Menorrhagia and its treatment with aminocaproic acid as assessed in a review by a group of randomly selected general practitioners. *Br. J. Clin. Pract.*, **31**, 14

Lithgow, D. M. and Politzer, W. M. (1977). Vitamin A in the treatment of menorrhagia. *S. Afr. Med. J.*, **51**, 191

Ludwig H. (1980). Intrauterinpessare: Veränderungen am Endometrium und am Pessar nach verschieden langer Liegezet in situ. *Verh. Dt. Ges. Pathol.*, **64**, 523

Ludwig, H. and Mehring, W. (1965). Zur Behandlung uteriner Blutungen mit Epsilon-Amino-capronsäure. *Fortschr. Med.*, **83**, 585

Ludwig, H., Metzger, H., Callies, R., Walx, K. A. and Kuppe, G. (1976). The tissue surface of the human endometrium after insertion of intrauterine contraceptive devices. In *SEM Proceedings, Workshop on SEM in Reproductive Biology*, p. 343. (Chicago: IIT Research Institute)

MacMath, I. F. (1973). Antifibrinolytic control of menorrhagia after IUD insertion. *The Practitioner*, **210**, 417

Melander, B., Gliniecki, G., Granstrand, B. and Hanshoff, G. (1965). Biochemistry and toxicology of Amikapron; the antifibrinolytically active isomer of AMCA. *Acta Pharmacol. Toxicol.*, **22**, 340

Morse, K. N., Peterson, W. F. and Allen, S. T. (1966). Endometrial effects of an intrauterine contraceptive device. *Obstet. Gynecol.*, **28**, 323

Moyer, D. L. and Mishell, D. R., Jr. (1971). Reactions of human endometrium to the intrauterine foreign body. II. Long-term effects on the endometrial histology and cytology. *Am. J. Obstet. Gynecol.*, **111**, 66

Moyer, D. L. and Shaw, S. T., Jr. (1973). Intrauterine devices: biochemical action. In Hafez, E. S. S. and Evans, T. N. (eds.) *Human Reproduction, Conception and Contraception*, p. 309. (New York: Harper & Row)

Moyer, D. T., Shaw, S. T., Jr., Fu, J., Hohman, W. R. and Thompson, R. S. (1978). Preclinical intrauterine contraception. In Ludwig, H. and Tauber, P. F. (eds.) *Human Fertilization*, p. 226. (Stuttgart: Thieme Verlag)

Nilsson, I. M. (1975). Local fibrinolysis as a mechanism for hemorrhage. *Thrombos. Diathes. Haemorrh. (Stutt.)*, **34**, 623

Nilsson, I. M. and Björkman, S. E. (1965). Experiences with epsilon-aminocaproic acid (EACA) in the treatment of profuse menstruation. *Acta Med. Scand.*, **177**, 445

Nilsson, L. and Rybo, G. (1967). Treatment of menorrhagia with an antifibrinolytic agent, tranexamic acid (AMCA). A double blind study. *Acta Obstet. Gynecol. Scand.*, **46**, 572

Nilsson, L. and Rybo, G. (1971). Treatment of menorrhagia. *Am. J. Obstet. Gynecol.*, **110**, 713

Piotrow, T., Rinehart, W. and Schmidt, J. C. (1979). IUDs – Update on safety, effectiveness and research. *Population Reports*, Series B, No. 3

Ragab, M. I. and Thomas, M. N. (1976). The use of tranexamic acid (AMCA) in IUDs as an anti-bleeding agent. *Int. J. Gynecol. Obstet.*, **14**, 137

Rendina, G. M. and Patrono, D. (1976). The use of a biological preparation in the treatment of some gynecological diseases. *Curr. Med. Res. Opin.*, **4**, 151

Rybo, G. (1966). Plasminogen activators in the endometrium. II. Clinical Aspects. *Acta Obstet. Gynaecol. Scand.*, **45**, 429

Rybo, G. (1978). The IUD and endometrial bleeding. *J. Reprod. Med.*, **20**, 175

Saksena, S. K. and Harper, M. J. K. (1974). Prostaglandin-mediated action of intrauterine devices: F-prostaglandins in the uterine horns of pregnant rabbits with unilateral intrauterine devices. *Fertil. Steril.*, **25**, 121

Schumacher, G. F. B. and Schill, W.-B. (1972). Radial diffusion in gel for microdetermination of enzyme II. Plasminogen activator, elastase and non-specific proteases. *Analyt. Biochem.*, **48**, 9

Schumacher, G. F. B. and Zaneveld, L. J. D. (1974). Proteinase inhibitors in human cervical mucus and their *in vitro* interactions with human acrosin. In Fritz, H., Tschesche, H., Greene, L. J. and Truscheit E. (eds.) *Proteinase Inhibitors*, p. 178. (Berlin: Springer Verlag)

Shaw, S. T., Jr., Cihak, R. W. and Moyer, D. L. (1970). Fibrin proteolysis in the monkey uterine cavity: Variations with and without IUD. *Nature*, **228**, 1097

Shaw, S. T., Jr., Moyer, D. L., Aaronson, D. E., Underwood, J. and Forino, R. V., (1975). Intrauterine medication with epsilon aminocaproic acid. Effect on Rhesus monkeys wearing intrauterine devices. *Contraception*, **11**, 395

Tauber, P. F. (1979a). Biochemical components of the endometrium. In Beller, F. and Schumacher, G. F. B., (eds.) *The Biology of the Fluids of the Female Genital Tract*, p. 131. (New York: Elsevier North-Holland)

Tauber, P. F. (1979b). Uterine Blutungen bei intrauteriner Kontrazeption: Pathophysiologie und Therapie. *Med. Welt*, **30**, 1547

Tauber, P. F. and Wolf, A. S. (1975). Beeinflussung unerwünschter IUD-Nebenwirkungen durch lokale Antifibrinolyse. Presented at the *Spring Meeting of the Upper Rhine Society of Obstetrics and Gynecology*, Ulm, West Germany

Tauber, P. F., Herting, W., Kurz, E. and Feichter, G. E. (1977a). Lokale Proteinase-Inhibitor-Konzentration im uterinen Sekret bei Intrauterinspiralen (IUD) in situ. *Arch. Gynecol.*, **224**, 32

Tauber, P. F., Wolf, A. S., Herting, W. and Zaneveld, L. J. D. (1977b). Hemorrhage induced by intrauterine devices: Control by local proteinase inhibition. *Fertil. Steril.*, **28**, 1375

Tauber, P. F., Herting, W., Zaneveld, L. J. D., Propping, D. and Ludwig, H. (1978). Intrauterine contraception and its side-effects: Effects of local proteinase inhibition. In Ludwig, H. and Tauber, P. F. (eds.) *Human Fertilization*, p. 261. (Stuttgart: Thieme Verlag)

Tauber, P. F., Werling, E., Klöppel, A. and Ludwig, H. (1979). Ergebnisse einer Blutungsprophylaxe mit Fibrinolyse-Inhibitoren bei intrauteriner Kontrazeption. *Arch. Gynecol.*, **228**, 637

Trévoux, R. (1977). Une indication inédite du sulpiride: Les Hémorragies utérines fonctionelles. *J. Gynecol. Obstet. Biol. Reprod.*, **6**, 1133

Umezawa, H. (1972). *Enzyme Inhibitors of Microbial Origin*. (Baltimore, Md.: University Park Press)

Unkeless, J. C., Gordon, S. and Reich, E. (1974). Secretion of plasminogen activator by stimulated macrophages. *J. Exp. Med.*, **139**, 834

Vermylen, J., Verhaegen-Declercq, M. L., Verstraete, M. and Fierens, F. (1968). A double-blind study of the effect of tranexamic acid in essential menorrhagia. *Thromb. Diathes. Haematol.*, **20**, 583

Weström, L. and Bengtsson, L. P. (1970). Effect of tranexamic acid (AMCA) in menorrhagia with intrauterine contraceptive devices. *J. Reprod. Med.*, **5**, 154

Wolf, A. S., Tauber, P. F. and Zaneveld, L. J. D. (1975). Decrease of IUD-associated side effects through intrauterine application of proteinase inhibitors. *Reproduccion*, **2**, 333

Yang, S.-L., Zaneveld, L. J. D. and Schumacher, G. F. B. (1976). Effect of serum proteinase inhibitors on the fertilizing capacity of rabbit spermatozoa. *Fertil. Steril.*, **27**, 577

Ylikorkala, O., Kaippila, A. and Siljauder, M. (1978). Antiprostaglandin therapy in prevention of side-effects of intrauterine contraceptive devices. *Lancet*, **2**, 393

Zaneveld, L. J. D., Polakoski, K. L., Robertson, R. T. and Williams, W. L. (1971). Tryspin inhibitors and fertilization. In *Proceedings of an International Research Conference on Proteinase Inhibitors, Munich, 1970*, p. 236. (Berlin: de Gruyter)

Zipper, J., Medel, M., Pastene, L. and Rivera, M. (1969). Intrauterine instillation of chemical cytotoxic agents for tubal sterilization and treatment of functional metrorrhagias. *Int. J. Fertil.*, **14**, 280

11
IUDs and pregnancy

G. S. BERGER AND L. G. KEITH

Pregnancy with an IUD *in situ* has long been recognized as a complication of intrauterine contraception. Early reports on IUDs in modern medical practice observed that ectopic as well as intrauterine pregnancies occurred with the IUD *in situ* (Grafenberg, 1929). Since then, the process by which medicated and non-medicated IUDs exert their antifertility effects has been studied extensively in laboratory animals as well as in the human. Nonetheless, the precise mechanism of action of the IUD remains unknown. In this regard, there appear to be considerable differences not only among animal species but also between animals and humans.

The reasons why IUDs do not consistently prevent either intrauterine or ectopic pregnancy have been reviewed elsewhere in detail (Edelman *et al.*, 1979). In this chapter the risks of pregnancies, begun with the IUD *in situ*, the outcomes of these pregnancies, and the effects of IUD use on subsequent fertility will be considered.

IUD PREGNANCY RATES

General comments

Of the many types of IUD that have been evaluated clinically in the USA, only five are commercially available: the Lippes Loop, Saf-T-Coil, Cu-7, Tatum-T, and Progestasert. For these IUDs, Table 11.1 shows the net cumulative 1-year life table pregnancy rates per 100 women based on product information supplied by the manufacturers of the IUDs or from material referenced by the manufacturers.

Although presently not available in the USA, the Multiload IUD is widely used in Europe and other parts of the world. Data from one multi-clinic study including 2782 women has indicated low event rates, especially for pregnancy, when compared with the devices shown in Table 11.1. The 1-year net cumulative life table rates per 100 women for pregnancy, expulsion, and medical removals were 0.5, 2.2, and 5.4, respectively (Thiery

Table 11.1 One-year net cumulative life table pregnancy rates per 100 women for IUDs commercially available in the USA

IUD	*No. of insertions*	*Pregnancy rates*
Lippes Loop[a]		
Size A	1015	5.3
Size B	1305	3.4
Size C	3489	3.0
Size D	7553	2.7
Saf-T-Coil (all sizes)[b]	NS[c]	2.4
Cu-7 (Gravigard)[d]:		
Nulliparas	NS[e]	1.6
Multiparas	NS	1.9
Cu-T-200B (Tatum-T)[d]:		
Nulliparas	NS	2.1
Multiparas	NS	3.0
Progestasert[f]		
Nulliparas	7614	2.6
Multiparas		1.8

[a] Ortho Pharmaceutical Corporation, Raritan, N.J., USA
[b] Schmidt Laboratories, Little Falls, N.J., USA
[c] Not stated; 4231 women completed 12 months of use
[d] Searle Laboratories, Chicago, Ill., USA
[e] Not Stated; 11 852 women completed 12 months of Cu-7 use; 8232 women completed 12 months of Cu-T-200 use
[f] Alza Pharmaceuticals, Palo Alto, Ca. USA

et al., 1978). Before a final assessment of the Multiload performance can be made, however, additional large-scale, multi-clinic, and independent trials will be required.

Problems in data interpretation

It is important to recognize that the pregnancy rates shown in Table 11.1 are average rates which have been derived from many studies, and that the results from any particular study may differ considerably from this average rate. There are a number of reasons why divergent results can be expected from studies of the same type of IUD evaluated among different populations of women. They include:

(1) the fecundability of the population (Tietze, 1968);
(2) the age/parity composition of the population (Snowden *et al.*, 1977); and
(3) Social-cultural factors affecting the frequency and timing of intercourse during the menstrual cycle (Edelman *et al.*, 1979).

The pregnancy rates given in a study can also be influenced by the methods used to collect the study data and the methods used to evaluate and report the study results. For example, studies in which there is an inadequate follow-up of subjects either grossly underestimate or overestimate the actual pregnancy rate depending on whether women who become pregnant return to the clinic or seek treatment and/or advice elsewhere. A more complete discussion of the biases that may result from the use of an inappropriate study design and analytical procedures has been presented elsewhere (Edelman *et al.*, 1979).

THE RISKS OF ECTOPIC PREGNANCY

General observations

Ever since it was reported that four (17.4%) out of 23 women who became pregnant with a Lippes Loop *in situ* had ectopic pregnancies (Lippes, 1965), questions have been raised as to whether the IUD *causes* ectopic pregnancy and whether it is effective in preventing ectopic pregnancy.

By 1970, it was thought that non-medicated IUDs were highly effective in preventing intrauterine pregnancies, less effective in preventing tubal pregnancies, and afforded no protection against ovarian pregnancies (Lehfeldt *et al.*, 1970). It was also believed that the increase in the incidence of ectopic pregnancy observed in the UK in the early 1970s probably was associated with increased use of IUDs (Beral, 1975). Investigators in Turku, Finland, believed that the increased incidence of ectopic pregnancy was due to the IUD (Erkkola and Liukko, 1977). Other workers in the UK found a higher risk of ectopic contraceptive users (Vessey *et al.*, 1979). On the other hand, data from the USA suggested that the use of IUDs was not a major factor contributing to the increased incidence of ectopic pregnancy (Sivin, 1979).

Critical review of the literature

To our knowledge, there is no evidence in the literature to support the contention that the IUD *causes* ectopic pregnancy. The issue is really one of how effective is the IUD in preventing ectopic pregnancy. The notion that IUDs cause ectopic pregnancy is probably a result of misinterpretation of reported data and a result of faulty studies and analyses to assess the risks of ectopic pregnancies (Edelman *et al.*, 1979).

Epidemiologic studies such as that of Beral (Beral, 1975), generally have failed to consider all factors that might affect the incidence of ectopic pregnancy. Since the prevalence of IUD use is fairly well known and the risks of pregnancy while using an IUD also are well documented, it may be tempting to attribute changes in the incidence of ectopic pregnancies to increases in the reported use of IUDs. Unfortunately, those epidemiological studies which favor this relationship have failed to evaluate the effects of the venereal disease epidemic of the past decade on ectopic pregnancies. The causal relationship between pelvic inflammatory disease and subsequent risk of ectopic pregnancy has long been established and cannot be overlooked.

The prevalent belief that IUDs cause ectopic pregnancy probably stems from the observation that the risk of ectopic pregnancy to the IUD user who becomes pregnant may be 5–10 times higher than for the non-contraceptive user who becomes pregnant. From the following model, one can see that this indeed is an erroneous conclusion. Assume that one out of 80 women who become pregnant is at risk of an ectopic pregnancy and that in a group of 100 non-contraceptive users, 80 will become pregnant. Out of this group there will be 79 intrauterine and one (1.25%) ectopic pregnancies. In a similar group of 100 women using IUDs, four pregnancies would be expected, if it is assumed that the IUD is effective in preventing 96% of all pregnancies. If the IUD were completely ineffective in preventing ectopic pregnancy, one would still expect one ectopic pregnancy in the group of 100 users. Thus in the IUD group there would be three intrauterine pregnancies and one (25%) ectopic pregnancy.

Table 11.2 Ectopic pregnancy rates for different IUDs

IUD	*Woman-months of use*	*Ectopic pregnancy rates/ 100 woman-years*
Cu-7	157 625	0.04
Cu-T	132 432	0.05
Non-medicated	343 365	0.12
Progestasert	126 800	0.40

From *FDA Drug Bulletin* (1979)

In fact, IUDs probably do prevent some ectopic pregnancies and some types of IUDs may be more effective in preventing ectopic pregnancy than others (Table 11.2). The data in Table 11.2 were derived originally from many different sources and provide only a partial indication of the relative risk of ectopic pregnancy for different types of IUDs. To evaluate these relative risks more accurately, one would also have to consider the proportions of women in the different studies who had any of the known risk factors which predispose them to ectopic pregnancy *before* insertion of the IUD. Among these are PID and prior ectopic pregnancy. In reality, the true effectiveness of the IUD in preventing ectopic pregnancy may indeed be related to the mechanism through which the IUD exerts its antifertility effects rather than the other factors, but the question remains unclear (Edelman *et al.*, 1979).

There is no uniform agreement as to whether the risk of ectopic pregnancy increases with the duration of IUD use. Data from the Oxford Family Planning Association contraceptive study do not indicate any increased risk of ectopic pregnancy with increasing duration of IUD use (Vessey *et al.*, 1979). In that study, the risk of ectopic pregnancy remained constant with duration of IUD use, at about 1.2 $(1000 \text{ women})^{-1} \text{year}^{-1}$. On the other hand, data from the Population Council based on their extensive evaluations of the Cu-T IUDs indicate a significant increase in the risk of ectopic pregnancy with duration of IUD use (from 0.63 per 1000 women during the first year of use to 3.68 per 1000 women during the fourth year of use). This latter rate is similar to or lower than that of the non-contraceptor.

Summary

The cumulative evidence from the extensive literature on intrauterine contraception provides no evidence for any causal relationship between IUD use and ectopic pregnancy. The IUD user who becomes pregnant is at a higher risk of ectopic pregnancy, but in absolute terms this risk is lower than the risk of ectopic pregnancy in the non-contraceptive user who becomes pregnant.

THE OUTCOME OF INTRAUTERINE PREGNANCIES

General observations

It is unlikely that the near future will see the development of an IUD that has a zero pregnancy rate. It is more likely that regardless of device type, about 2–4% of IUD users will become pregnant with their IUD *in situ*. Assuming a worldwide prevalence of 35 million IUD users, one can expect that from 0.7 to 1.4 million women will become pregnant while using an IUD. Even though all of these pregnancies may be unwanted, not all women have immediate or easy access to legal abortion and elective termination of pregnancy. The outcomes of their pregnancies thus are of concern to the women and their physicians.

Spontaneous abortion

Accumulated data from the IUD literature indicates that women who either do not have their IUDs removed or who do not expel their IUD after conception has occurred are at about twice the risk of a spontaneous abortion compared with women who expel their IUDs or have them removed (Table 11.3). Stillbirth rates, on the other hand, are about the same for both groups of women. The mechanisms by which the IUD increases the likelihood of a spontaneous abortion are unknown. No evidence has been presented to indicate that any of the commercially available IUDs in the USA (Cu-7, Cu-T-200, Lippes Loop, Progestasert, Saf-T-Coil) are associated with different rates of spontaneous abortion.

Table 11.3 Outcome of pregnancies with an IUD in situ

	Outcome of pregnancy		
	Live birth (%)	*Stillbirth (%)*	*Spontaneous abortion (%)*
IUD not removed after conception	46.1	1.0	52.9
IUD removed or expelled after conception	75.5	1.0	23.5

From: Edelman *et al.* (1979)

Septic spontaneous abortion

There are inadequate data to assess the risks of septic spontaneous abortion among IUD users who become pregnant with the IUD *in situ* (Edelman *et al.*, 1979). Reports on serious septic complications among IUD users who became pregnant have led to an increased awareness of the risks to any IUD user who becomes pregnant with an IUD *in situ*. Current medical practice dictates that the IUD be removed immediately if the woman is pregnant and has an IUD *in situ*. If she declines to have her IUD removed, the patient must be informed of her increased risks of a spontaneous abortion and the life-threatening complications that may develop if there is concurrent sepsis.

The Center for Disease Control compiled data on septic spontaneous abortion deaths in the USA from 1972 to 1975. In the period 1972 to mid-1974, there were 42 deaths in association with septic spontaneous abortion, 17 of which occurred to women using IUDs. In the period from mid-1974 to 1975, there were 20 septic spontaneous abortion deaths; none of these women were IUD users (Cates *et al.*, 1977). From 1975 to 1979, two septic spontaneous abortion deaths were reported in association with the use of IUDs (Cates, unpublished observations). This decline in IUD-related septic spontaneous abortion deaths is probably related to the awareness by medical personnel for the need to remove the IUD immediately in women who become pregnant.

Congenital malformations

A concern of any woman who elects to carry to term a pregnancy begun with the IUD *in situ* is the possibility of a congenital malformation of the fetus. The only study which specifically evaluated the association between IUD use and congenital abnormalities found no increased risk of congenital abnormalities among the offspring of women who reported that they conceived with an IUD *in situ*, compared with women who reported that they did not have an IUD *in situ* at conception (Layde *et al.*, 1979).

Many congenital abnormalities go undetected. Pregnancies are often spontaneously or electively aborted before any abnormalities can be recognized. Even with more advanced pregnancies (i.e. late first or early second trimester), only gross abnormalities may be recognized.

At present, there is no evidence to indicate any increased risk of congenital abnormalities for women who become pregnant while using any type of available IUD.

FERTILITY AFTER IUD DISCONTINUATION

Since the IUD is not intended to be a permanent method of contraception, many women who discontinue IUD use do so to become pregnant. For this reason, it is important that the IUD not have any permanent antifertility effects and that the interval from discontinuation of IUD use to pregnancy be as short as possible.

Table 11.4 Pregnancy rates at 1 year after IUD discontinuation

Reference	*No. of subjects*	*IUD(s)*	*1-Year pregnancy rate*
Alza Corporation (1977)	154	Progestasert	76.0[a]
Ellinas (1977)	NS	Types not specified	96.8%
Sivin and Stern (1979)	420	Copper-T (all models)	78.1[a]
Sakurabayashi (1966)	35	Polyethylene ring	80.0%
Tietze (1968)	611	Lippes Loop, Margulies Spiral, Birnberg Bow, Steel Ring, Saf-T-Coil	77.0%
Kaye *et al.* (1977)	36	Lippes Loop, Saf-T-Coil, Dalkon Shield Cu-7	88.9%

[a] Net cumulative life table rate per 100 women
NS = Not Stated

About 80–90% of the women who discontinue IUD use to get pregnant will conceive within 12 months (Table 11.4). The pregnancy rates appear to be independent of the type of IUD used. Variations in the rates shown in Table 11.4 probably reflect the different methods used to report fertility rates, the adequacy of follow-up, and the fertility of the group of women under study. The limitation to the studies enumerated in Table 11.4 is that they give the subsequent fertility of a selected group of women who state that they want their IUDs removed to become pregnant. The fertility of women who discontinue IUD use for non-voluntary reasons, e.g. removal for bleeding and/or pain or infection, has not yet been evaluated.

The proportion of women who become pregnant within 1 year after discontinuation of IUD use appears to be higher than the comparable rate for women who discontinue oral or injectable contraceptives and similar to the rate for women who discontinue barrier contraceptives (Ellinas, 1977; Vessey *et al.*, 1976). The outcome of pregnancies begun after IUD discontinuation has not yet been evaluated extensively. In one study no differences were found in the outcome of pregnancies between women who stopped using their IUDs, those who stopped taking oral contraceptives, and those who stopped using barrier methods (Vessey *et al.*, 1976).

CONCLUDING REMARKS

There is no IUD associated with a pregnancy rate of zero. The generally accepted risk of pregnancy is about 2–4 pregnancies per 100 women-years. Intrauterine and ectopic pregnancy are both recognized as hazards associated with the use of any IUD. Since the development of an IUD which is 100% effective in preventing pregnancy is unlikely, it is important to recognize pregnancy-related complications of IUD use.

Acknowledgments

Supported in part by The Center For The Advancement Of Reproductive Health, Chapel Hill, NC, and The Charles A. Fields Medical Foundation, Chicago.

References

Alza Corporation (1977). *The Progestasert. Intrauterine Progesterone Contraceptive System Release Rated 65 μg/Day Progesterone for One Year.* (Palo Alto, Ca.: Alza Product Information

Beral, V. (1975). An epidemiologic study of recent trends in ectopic pregnancy. *Br. J. Obstet. Gynaecol.*, **82**, 775

Cates, W., Grimes, D. A., Ory, H. W. and Tyler, C. W. (1977). Publicity and the public health: The elimination of IUD-related abortion deaths. *Family Planning Perspectives*, **9**, 138

Edelman, D. A., Berger, G. S. and Keith, L. (1979). *Intrauterine Devices and Their Complications.* (Boston, Ma.: G. K. Hall)

Ellinas, S. P. (1977). Experience with medroxyprogesterone acetate (Depo-Provera) as an injectable contraceptive. *Int. J. Gynaecol. Obstet.*, **15**, 145

Erkkola, R. and Liukko, P. (1977). Intrauterine device and ectopic pregnancy. *Contraception*, **16**, 569

FDA Drug Bulletin (1979). Progestasert IUD and ectopic pregnancy. *FDA Drug Bull.*, **8**, 37

Grafenberg, E. (1929). Die intrauterine method der konceptionsurhusdtung. In *Intrauterine Contraceptive Rings: History and Statistical Appraisal. Third Congress of the World League for Sexual Reform*, International Congress Series, No. 54, (Amsterdam: Excerpta Medica)

Kaye, B. M., Reaney, B. V., Kaye, D. L. and Edelman, D. A. (1977). Longterm safety and use-effectiveness of intrauterine devices. *Fertil. Steril.*, **28**, 937

Layde, P. M., Goldberg, M. F., Safra, M. J. and Oakley, G. P. (1979). Failed intrauterine device contraception and limb reduction deformities: A case control study. *Fertil. Steril.*, **31**, 18

Lehfeldt, H., Tietze, C. and Gorstein, F. (1970). Ovarian pregnancy and the intrauterine device. *Am. J. Obstet. Gynecol.*, **108**, 1005

Lippes, J. (1965). Contraceptive with intrauterine plastic loops. *Am. J. Obstet. Gynecol.*, **93**, 1024

Sakurabayashi, M. (1966). Experience with polyethylene ring: 1955–1965, Part 1. *Yokohama Med. Bull.*, **17**, 91

Sivin, I. (1979). Copper-T IUD use and ectopic pregnancy rates in the United States. *Contraception*, **19**, 151

Sivin, J. and Stern, J. (1979). Long-acting, more effective Copper-T IUDs: A summary of U.S. experience, 1970–1975. *Stud. Family Planning*, **10**, 263

Snowden, R., Williams, M. and Hawkins, D. (1977). *The IUD: A Practical Guide.* (London: Croom Helm)

Thiery, M., van der Pas, H., van Os, W. A. A., Dombrowicz, N., MacDonald, J. S., Haspels, A. A., Drogendijk, A. C., van Kets, H. and Boogers, W. (1978). Three years' experience with the ML Cu250, a new copper-wired intrauterine contraceptive device. *Adv. Planning Parenthood.*, **13**, 35

Tietze, C. (1968). Fertility after discontinuation of intrauterine and oral contraception. *Int. J. Fertil.*, **13**, 385

Vessey, M., Doll, R., Peto, R., Johnson, B. and Wiggins, P. (1976). A longterm follow-up study of women using different methods of contraception – an interim report. *J. Biosoc. Sci.*, **8**, 373

Vessey, M. P., Yeates, D. and Flavel, R. (1979). Risk of ectopic pregnancy and duration of use of an intrauterine device. *Lancet*, **2**, 501

12
Psychological aspects of IUD use

B. BOURGEOIS

The acceptance of an IUD depends on four factors: (1) the type of IUD; (2) the woman's personality; (3) the doctor's personality; and (4) the context of the prescription, IUD insertion, and follow-up. This last point reflects the doctor–patient relationship, which is essential to medical psychology and too often forgotten or assumed to be too evident to require discussion (Balint, 1957).

To establish a satisfactory experience with contraception, the introduction must be informative so the woman feels secure with her decision. The physician should explain all the available choices, insertion procedure, and the pro's and con's. The future success of contraception depends on technological progress. A greater understanding will promote a better psychological standpoint. Improving the training of doctors in this specialized field will enable this doctor–patient relationship to be more successful. Differences between one clinical center and another are often greater than the differences in performance between two different devices (Population Reports, 1975). Differences are also apparent between any two doctors.

Insertion may create some pain or discomfort. Little information is available on the intensity and nature of this pain (Massay *et al.*, 1974). A comparison of IUD insertion in 24 women taking naproxen, an analgesic, and 26 women taking placebo was made. Pain was as common in the two groups at insertion and immediately after insertion, but more common in the placebo group after 1 hour.

The psychological factors governing the perception of pain are becoming better understood and are being given greater consideration (Melzach, 1973). The factors consist of: anxiety, superstitions, mental attitudes, personality, mood of the patient (mild depression increases the sensation of pain), and the focusing of the patient's attention. Anxiety lowers the pain threshold and increases muscular tension, which may make insertion difficult. Anxiety is created by not informing the patient of detailed procedure, the expected pain, and its duration. A reassuring manner is essential.

IUD REMOVAL DUE TO PAIN AND BLEEDING

Attitudes, experience, and ability of the practitioner inserting the IUD often influences the rate of IUD removal. The rate of removal falls from 9% (when the doctor is learning the technique) to 2.5% when the doctor has become familiar with the method (Bernard, 1971). Insertion is then more rapidly and easily performed. Time gained may be used for the psychological preparation of the patient. The confidence of the practitioner is quite perceptible to the client. Fewer side-effects exist when the doctor's approach is more informal (Snowden *et al.*, 1973). The degree of attentiveness of the attending doctor was also found to have a marked effect on the bleeding–pain removal rate (Lippes, 1967). Single-doctor clinics were found to do appreciably better than multi-doctor clinics (Bernard, 1971). The socio-economic condition is also important. Lower-class women were less likely to report bleeding for fear that the device would be removed (Wilson *et al.*, 1967). Women of higher economic status usually had an alternative contraceptive method and tolerated only a minimum of pain.

PSYCHOLOGICAL PREPARATION BEFORE INSERTION

Mental preparation of both doctor and patient, which is quite independent of the insertion skill, is very important (Bernard, 1971). The atmosphere surrounding a woman's first experience with an IUD often determines its ultimate acceptance. To develop acceptance, the practitioner should first be certain of the woman's wish and determination for contraception; in particular, for the IUD. A clear and understandable explanation of intrauterine contraception and insertion technique should be provided. Various techniques could be used on apprehensive patients, such as relaxation, hypnosis, music, or visual fixation on a picture. Friendly discussion before and during insertion will help the patient to relax and to be distracted. Since IUDs are easily forgotten once inserted, compared with a daily reminder to take the pill, the initial insertion period should be successfully administered.

THE PATIENT'S CHOICE IN CONTRACEPTION

Most women usually expect the gynecologist to determine which contraceptive method they should use. Only a few women are enthusiastic about selecting a contraceptive method (Kinch, 1979). The patient's choice of a contraceptive method is influenced by the following six factors:

(1) Her attitude towards contraception.
(2) The physician's choice.
(3) Her assessment of risk from media information and knowledge of disasters occurring to friends.
(4) Her motivation and compliance for reliable contraception.
(5) Her previous experience with contraception.
(6) Her partner's experience.

SOCIAL FACTORS AND PERSONAL CHARACTERISTICS IN THE CHOICE OF CONTRACEPTIVE

Comparisons have been made between 772 pill acceptors and 582 IUD acceptors in 1354 women (Kingsley and McEwans, 1977). IUD users were more likely to be married, of high parity, to have had previous contraceptive experience, and to have had previous abortions. The pill acceptors were younger.

The necessity for obtaining contraception follows the following three phases:

(1) Sexually active adolescence and early adulthood (married and unmarried), with a need for a highly effective method without endangering future fertility.
(2) Family building period: spacing of birth rather than certainty of prevention is the goal; accidental pregnancies can occur.
(3) When the couple have completed the size of the family they intended to have highly effective control is needed again.

CONTRACEPTIVE PILL AND/OR IUD

Extensive literature on contraception is concerned mainly with oral contraception (OC) and often neglects the IUD, from emotional and psychological aspects. The greater use of the pill (in France at least three-quarters of women using modern contraception use the pill; one-quarter use an IUD) does not entirely explain this omission. Comparisons between the two methods are of interest.

Most double-blind studies for side-effects compare one method with the other. Like the pill, the IUD is an example of a modern and medical contraceptive method (i.e. one possessing safety, effectiveness, acceptability and reversibility). It is not directly associated with the sexual act. Unlike OC, the IUD is a local and mechanical method, without diffuse hormonal effect. The woman, the passive recipient, may forget about it after the initial insertion but the pill must be taken daily. Most women do, indeed, forget their IUD. So apparently, do the physicians and the researchers. Some have also insisted it is an abortifacient, confusing medical and ethical issues.

PSYCHOLOGICAL ASPECTS AND SIGNIFICANT CHARACTERISTICS OF THE IUD

The IUD is a type of prosthesis which modern medicine uses to modify a woman's physiology and improve the quality and comfort of her life. But in some cases it is not well incorporated into the body image. Some may unconsciously consider it a dangerous foreign body, 'a bad object', destructive, carcinogenic, even a 'sadic penis' or a pathological pregnancy – thus provoking relapse into former delusional or anxiety states observed in certain psychotics. It should be remembered that the prevalence of schizophrenia in the general population is at least 0.5%. So in every gynecologist's practice it is likely that there are several schizophrenics. Even more common are borderline or psychotic personalities who are sometimes frightened by every intrusive bodily procedure. Consequently, gynecologists should avoid forcing a woman into having a IUD inserted.

The emotional overtones and symbolic significance of this reversible sterilization have been greatly emphasized: the control of her body and desires with continual access to sexual pleasure free from risk of pregnancy leads to a changed role and status for the women in her relationship with men. It seems that intrapsychic, rather than interpersonal, conflicts ambivalent wishes, and outdated attitudes may prevent acceptance of the IUD. Some women retain an intense, unconscious desire to become pregnant, sometimes dissociated from the desire for a child or the maternal role. Occasionally, the risk or possibility of pregnancy is necessary for the woman to obtain pleasure. Finally, sexuality remains under the influence of social and moral reprobation and may be overcome with guilt.

There will be more former psychiatric patients amongst those women not tolerating an IUD than amongst those who are happy with the method. In a series of women not tolerating the IUD 65% experienced psychiatric difficulties, whereas only 5% having no problem with IUD had previously met a psychiatrist (King, 1967). Only 10–25% of women express continual complaints of side-effects such as bleeding, cramps, spontaneous expulsion, and occasionally – in moments of anger or crisis – pulling out the IUD themselves. The IUD is the only method of contraception which does not allow a woman to change her mind immediately, or on impulse. This is an intolerable constraint for some women. Their feminine role comes into conflict with their defensiveness, competitive tendencies, and feelings of resentment towards men. They become tense and unable to keep the IUD. On the other hand, since the IUD is relatively unconnected with sexual intercourse (inserted, then forgotten) this may cause less guilt than the pill. As with the pill, its effectiveness may excite feelings of frustration, depression, and loss of libido among the ambivalent personalities who have an unconscious desire for pregnancy and/or a baby when consciously and rationally they have chosen to use a contraceptive.

Those who are effective users of contraception have been characterized as mature, independent, self-reliant, secure, ambitious, decisive, and intelligent. They have a good self-image, assume responsibility with ease and confidence, carry accepted tasks to completion, control their impulsiveness, and have the capacity to tolerate frustration. They establish and appreciate long-range goals and have a capacity to establish good communication and usually good sexual adjustments with their partners. Success in life, in business, and in marriage correlates well with success in contraceptive usage.

In the very respectable *Comprehensive Textbook of Psychiatry* Sandberg (1975) described (apparently seriously and with the help of *MS* magazine) a series of vignettes of women who have chosen different methods of contraception:

'The user of an IUD is not as completely characterized as the others but is believed to be comfortable with her body, loving, masturbatory, and highly orgasmic. She is fully accepting of the mutuality, "messiness", and spontaneity of pleasurable sexual activity. She is accepting of pregnancy and childbirth and is neither repulsed nor fearful when considering them. She is not anxious in passivity and does not feel threatened by events and situations beyond her control.

'The woman who happily chooses and uses OCs is modern, active, opportunistic, ambitious, accepting of the new role of women, acquisitive, and desirous of freedom. Men, children, and other contraceptive methods are a restrictor of personal freedom and indulgence.

'They also restrict the pursuit of personal opportunities. However, her desire for freedom, control, and personal mastery over fate are in conflict with desires to be cared for and tended. But passivity is threatening. Although marriage may not be seen in that light, pregnancy and childbirth are. Personal control of a totally efficient contraceptive method relieves concerns of potential personal imprisonment in a stereotyped woman's role.

'The diaphragm user is considered independent, self-reliant, logical, career-oriented, and competitive with men. She likes to be in control of herself and her sexuality as well as the males in the world about her. She may feel superior to men and contemptuous of them, but at the same time she retains a need for romance, love, male attention, and approval. Her sexual responsivity may be quite variable, depending on her degree of need to control and her competitiveness in achieving the same abandon and pleasure as the man. She tends to be hypochondriacal and threatened by illness, symptoms, or potential body changes that she cannot control. The intauterine device and OC are feared in this light. The diaphragm is under her reassuring observation and direct control. It allows her to dictate the sexual scene, prevents any unbecoming, uncontrolled, and unstructured spontaneity and suits her work ethic.'

Evidently, for Sandberg, women using traditional methods of contraception or those not using contraception are irresponsible, immature, retarded . . .

THE PHYSICIAN

Modern contraception is a medical technique. The husband has lost the initiative for birth control. Another partner intervenes: the physician, who plays a major role. The pill is seen as a medication and IUD insertion as an operation. The woman expects the doctor to decide about contraception or at least to give advice or approval. This change in the doctor–patient relationship (where a healthy woman prescribes for herself) may lead to problems of professional identity with reactionary refusals to comply with women's requests or misuse of the doctor's power, especially where adolescents are concerned. The need for respectability has led many gynecologists in France, for example, to adhere to restrictive practices, considering nulliparity an absolute contraindication to the IUD.

To be responsible for women's contraception implies an ideological and ethical stance on the part of the physician. That is also why gynecologists insist on the positive psychological aspects of the 'contraceptive revolution': woman's liberation, free access to sexual pleasure, and voluntary and responsible parenthood.

References

Balint, M. (1957). *The Doctor, His Patient, and the Illness.* (London: Pitman Medical)

Barwin, B. N. and Gosselin, J. Y. (1979). Psychological factors: counselling and motivation of the IUD patient. In Hafez, E. S. E. and van Os, W. A. A. (eds.) *Medicated IUDs and Polymeric Delivery Systems*

Bernard, R. P. (1970). IUD performance patterns - a 1970 world view. *Int. J. Gynecol. Obstet.*, **8**, 926

Bernard, R. P. (1971). Factors governing IUD performance. *Am. J. Public Health.*, **61**, 559

Bourgeois, M. (1980). Aspects medicopsychiatriques de la contraception moderne. *Bordeaux Med.*, **13**, 1285

Kinch, R. A. (1979). The patients' choice in contraception. *Int. J. Gynecol. Obstet.*, **16**, 561

Kingsley, S. and McEwans, J. (1977). Social factors in the choice of contraception method: a comparison of first clinic attenders accepting oral contraceptive with those accepting intrauterine devices. *J. Biosoc. Sci.*, **9**, 153

Pasini, W. (1971). Le desir de grossesse, fil d'Ariane de la gynecologie psychosomatique *Med. Hyg.*, **29**, 1

Pasini, W. (1974a). *Sexualite et Gynecologie Psychosomatique*, Vol. 1, p. 23. (Paris: Mabbon)

Pasini, W. (1974b). *Desir d'enfant et Contraception,* Vol. 1, p. 140. (Paris: Casterman)

Population Reports (1975). Series B, No. 2. January. Population Information Program,

Reading, A. E. and Newton, J. R. (1977). Psychological factors in IUD use. A review. *J. Biosoc. Sci.,* **9**, 317

Sandberg, E. C. (1975). Psychological aspects of contraception. In Freedman, A. M., Kaplan, H. T. and Sadock, B. J. (eds.) *Comprehensive Textbook of Psychiatry,* p. 1487. (Baltimore, Md.: Williams and Wilkins)

Snowden, R., Eckstein, P. and Hawkins, D. (1973). Social and medical factors in the use and effectiveness of IUD. *J. Biosoc. Sci.,* **5**, 31

(1979) *Regulation de la Fecondite, Bilan et Perspectives,* Colloque, Vol. 1. (Paris: INSERM)

Par[illegible]

IUDs AND FAMILY PLANNING

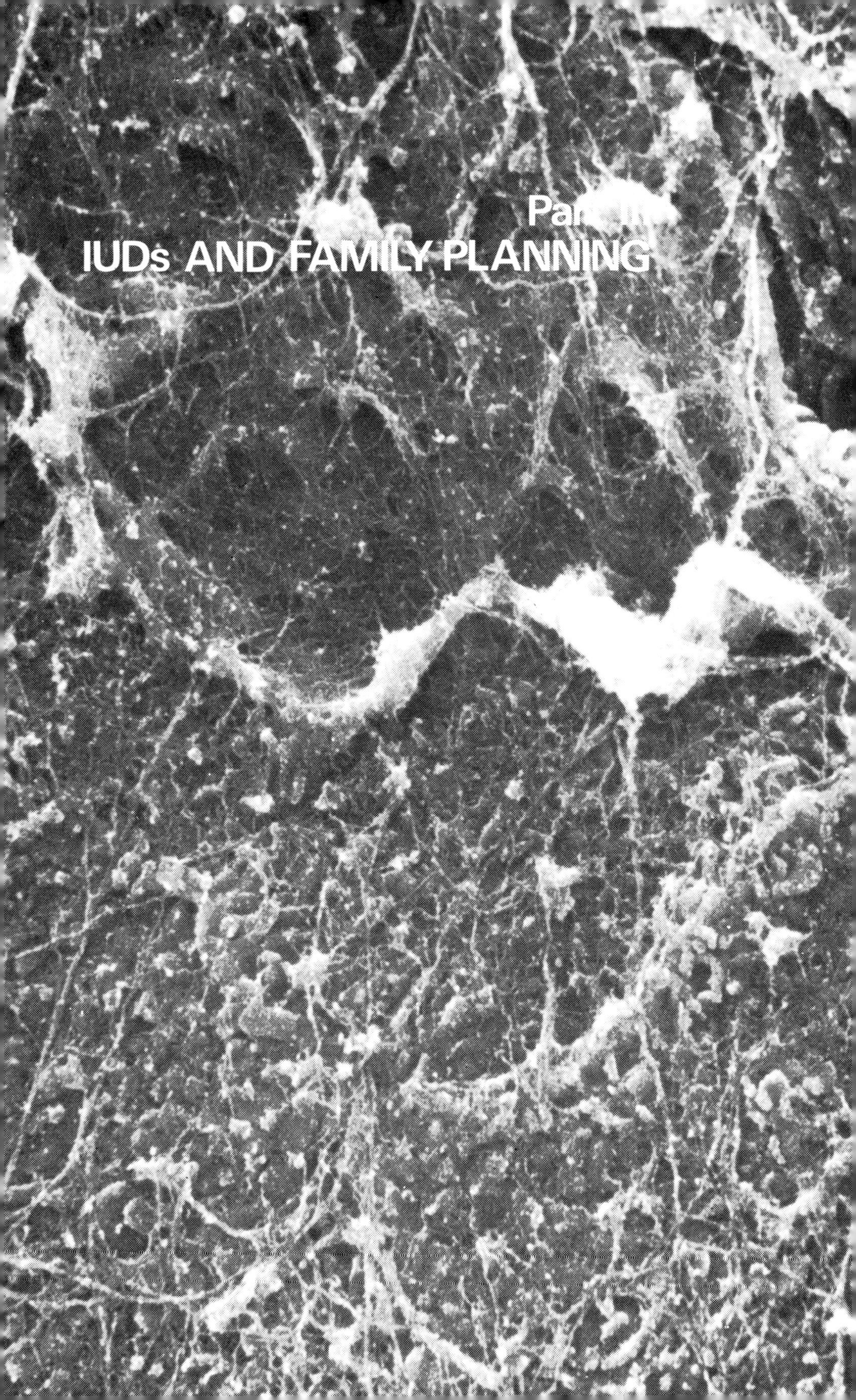

13
Role of IUDs in contraception throughout the world

M. LEVRIER

Empirical means to reduce fertility led to various abortive practices. Modern contraception, introduced in the 1960s by oral contraceptives (OCs) and IUDs, has provided couples with safer family planning opportunities. Current attempts at controlling male fertility have not yet yielded a satisfactory method of contraception (e.g. inhibition of gonadotrophins by cotton-seed derivates largely tested in China). More than 50% of the 4.5 billion world population are female. The estimated number of women risking pregnancy is about 500 million, 200 million of whom use some form of contraceptive method. Most women in countries with high birth rates (e.g. India, Indonesia, Brazil, Bangladesh, Nigeria, and Mexico) do not practice birth control. In more developed areas (e.g. North America and Western Europe), most women use contraception.

There are over 50 million IUD users (40 million in China alone), 55 million OC users, and over 30 million condom users. Nearly 90 million males or females are sterilized. Sterilization, for contraceptive purpose, is forbidden in France but allowed in other countries (e.g. USA, UK, Canada, India, and The Netherlands).

In developing countries, the IUD is used for family planning. In industrialized countries OCs are widely used, yet are often challenged by other methods, including the IUD. In North America and Western Europe, IUD use varies: 20% of women in Finland and Sweden use the IUD, 11% of women in France, 9% in Denmark, and only 3% in Italy. In the USA, 69% of all women practice contraception, 7% of whom are IUD users. In developing countries, Governments – supported by international bodies – are introducing birth control. The IUD is chosen for those women unable to practice family planning owing to natural improvidence, constraint aversion, poor education, or religious constraints.

IUD use further develops according to the number of pregnancies. Of those women who required replacement of their first IUD, 67% chose to renew the IUD, whereas 2.4% chose OCs, 3% preferred a vaginal method, and a very small percentage requested sterilization. Of those women over age 30, 87% continued using the IUD. Of the various types of IUDs used, 78% of the women chose to renew the Copper-T and Multiload IUD, 67% chose the Gravigard, 65% chose Sterlys, 54% chose Progestasert, and 38% chose the inert Omga.

FRANCE

In France, 80% of all fertile women either practice contraception or are sterilized. Among the remaining 20%, some are already sterile and others are still planning pregnancy. Owing to the high percentage of fertile women seeking contraception, France is a leading nation in contraception.

ITALY

5.6% of the women take OCs and 3% use IUDs. Abortion is legal during the first trimester for health or social reasons only. One million abortions are performed yearly, mostly in a clandestine manner.

SPAIN

Since the new regime there are more contraceptive users. The traditional withdrawal method is still most popular (23%). OCs are used by 13% of the female population and only 1% use IUDs. Being a Roman Catholic society, Spain still considers IUDs as abortive agents. Abortion and sterilization are not permitted.

PORTUGAL

Although abortion exists in Portugal, all other methods of contraception are used similarly to Spain. Family planning centers offer OCs, pessaries, and injectable progestagens.

UNITED KINGDOM

Before 1968 the condom was predominantly used, after which OCs and IUDs were promptly adopted. Between 1968 and 1975, use of modern contraception doubled. By 1975, OCs were used by 56% of the female population, 25% used the diaphragm, and 19% used IUDs. By 1973, 7% of the male and female fertile population had been sterilized (3% of men and 4% of women); by 1975, this figure rose to 12.5%. Because of unfavorable publications, OC use declined after 1975, yet still remains the most favorable method. Sterilization and abortion is becoming increasingly popular. Presently, 26% of the UK's fertile women population take OCs, 20% have partners who use condoms, 12% practice sterilization, and only 6% use IUDs.

SWEDEN AND NORWAY

OCs and IUDs are more popular methods of contraception. In Sweden,

IUDs are used by 20% of the fertile population and OCs are used by 32%. In Norway, IUDs are most popular and are used by 44% of all married women.

DENMARK

Denmark is one of the few industrialized countries willing to reduce the birth rate and is probably one of the most contraception adept nations in the world, since 92% of the fertile population practices contraception. OC use decreased from 28% in 1971 to 22% in 1977. Only 8% of the women use IUDs, yet their use is becoming more popular, even among younger women. Abortion and sterilization are permitted; however, men must be at least 25 years of age. Free abortions are becoming another common method of contraception.

FINLAND

The contraceptive situation in Finland is similar to that in Sweden (20% of the fertile population use OCs and 12.5% use an IUD).

BELGIUM

Although Belgium is another Roman Catholic country, 87% of all couples practice contraception. 29% of fertile women take OCs and 3% use IUDs.

THE NETHERLANDS

An over-population problem exists in this small country. Religious beliefs no longer interfere with contraceptive practice. 88% of married women use some method of contraception. OCs are used by 40–66% of the female population; condoms are used by the partners of 14% and IUDs are used by 4%. Sterilization is practiced mainly on older couples.

WEST GERMANY

A decrease in OC use has been seen since 1974; they are presently used by 28% of the population. IUD use is primarily practiced by women over 35 years of age.

USSR

Two or three different brands of OCs are available; they contain the heavier amount of hormones and are used minimally. Although accurate estimates are not obtainable, 2% of the 38 million married and fertile women use IUDs, which are inserted either after having an abortion, after age 25, or in women with high parity.

YUGOSLAVIA

Only 45% of the fertile women use contraception. The most popular method is male withdrawal. OCs are not easily available for economic reasons. Sterilization is permitted, but abortion is more readily practiced and the costs are reimbursed by the local social security system (in 1979, 300 000 abortions were reported).

USA

Since 1960 there has been a high birth rate decline and a widespread use of modern contraception. Abortion and sterilization are both practiced. Pill use increased from 1961 until 1968, then began to decline.

In 1977, 12% of fertile women used OCs and 20% of married women used OCs. A similar decline was seen with the IUD, which was due to the publicized adverse effects of both methods. Sterilization has become increasingly popular. Ten million American women are sterilized and one million men are vasectomized every year.

CANADA

Differences between the USA and Canada are few. In 1977, 19% of fertile women used OCs and 7% IUDs. Sterilization is steadily increasing. Only therapeutic abortion is permitted; however, many women cross the border into the USA to have abortions performed.

NEW ZEALAND AND AUSTRALIA

New Zealand is a developed country with large health care facilities. IUDs are widely used, yet 30–40% of women still use OCs. Throughout New Zealand and Australia, 10% of 2 million fertile women use IUDs.

JAPAN

Industrialization and birth decline run parallel, and the population growth rate is one of the lowest in the world. In 1977, 60% of fertile women practiced some contraception, including sterilization. 7% were IUD users and no more than 1–2% used OCs. There are one million Japanese women who wear IUDs. Since 1940, abortion has been permitted and is very popular. Sterilization is easily performed at least 50 000 times per year. IUDs were first investigated in the 1930s, yet their use was forbidden until 1974. Presently, two IUD models are locally made and distributed.

NORTH AFRICAN COUNTRIES

Morocco

The population doubles every 25 years. Family planning advice favors all methods. The IUD is preferred over OCs. A total of 6.2% of the women practice contraception, 1.3% of whom choose the IUD. Abortions are authorized only for the maintenance of the mother's health, but some are clandestinely performed. Sterilization is possible. Polygamy is vanishing.

Tunisia

A population increase exists; however, the Government has begun to enforce limitation. Marriages are being delayed; abortion is practiced, especially after the fifth child; family allowance money is reduced after the fourth child; polygamy has been abolished and family planning practices are free of charge. 22% of married women use contraception and 8% are IUD users, especially after the fourth child.

Algeria

Oral and injectable contraception are available; surgical sterilization is available only for women. IUDs are inserted by health co-workers and difficulties arise in multiparous uteri.

OTHER AFRICAN COUNTRIES

Contraception and abortion are not widely practiced in Central Africa. Little information is available.

In Nigeria, the IUD is preferred by 66% of young multiparous mothers. In Kenya, of 5% of women practicing contraception, 1% use an IUD. In Zaire, of 3% practicing contraception, one-third use the IUD.

In Mauritius, of 52% of couples practicing contraception, 25% abstain, 16% use the condom, and 1.5% of the women wear an IUD. There are an estimated 20 000 clandestine abortions per year.

THE ISLAMIC SOCIETY

The world Islamic population is 800 million, with one-half being younger than 15. The natural increase rate is 4%. Abortion is strictly forbidden, except in Tunisia before 4 months, unless for medical reasons, and after 4 months, unless the mother's life is in danger. Sterilization is banned in Korea. Islamic customs do not oppose family planning but people have been reluctant to practice contraception for quite a long time.

The progress made with contraception has created the belief that more and more people accept contraception throughout the world. The choice of the IUD is today the most favorable and will continue to be successful in the future.

In Sri Lanka, one-third of the women at risk of pregnancy practice contraception and 5% use the IUD. Of the 20% of the couples sterilized, most were female. 41 million women used an IUD in 1977 while 35% were taking OCs, which are available without prescription. There is no charge for contraception. Oral contraception is available for men. Abortion is legal.

CENTRAL AMERICA

In Mexico, of the 21% of women at risk of pregnancy practicing contraception, 8% are using IUDs. Since 1970, quarterly injectable contraception is offered for women above 30 or with four children. In Haiti and the Dominican Republic, about one-fifth of the women at risk of pregnancy practice contraception. IUD use is rare.

In Jamaica, of 42% of contraception users, 6.4% use the IUD.

In Cuba, all methods of contraceptive are available. Physicians insert IUDs and practice abortion. In Guatemala, of the 7.6% practicing contraception, 0.9% use the IUD. In Salvador and Nicaragua, of 4.3% using contraception, 3.8% are IUD users. In Costa Rica, 24% use injectable contraception, 5% use an IUD, 12% sterilization, and 9% have partners who use the condom. In Panama, 25% use sterilization (one-fifth of all women), 18% use injectable contraception, and 3–4% use the IUD.

SOUTH AMERICA

Considered as abortive, the IUD has been condemned by the Roman Catholic Church. Also, the insertion of a foreign body frightened women. Physicians, lacking practice, inserted few IUDs. Brazilian and Argentinian legislation have forbidden IUD sterilization. The birth rate in Argentina is not impressive and there are no birth control measures. Few women use an IUD.

In Brazil, IUD use is forbidden. In the most industrialized State, Sao Paulo, modern contraception is accepted. 73% of women at risk of pregnancy practice contraception, 1% use the IUD, and 8.4% use the pill. In Chile, of 70% practicing contraception, 18% use the IUD. In Colombia, of 42% of the women practicing contraception, 14% use an injectable contraceptive, 11% use an IUD, and 4% use sterilization. Male sterilization is widely practiced because it is cheap. In Venezuela, 88% of the women practicing contraception use the IUD, 10% the pill, and 4% sterilization. In Ecuador, only 9% of the women at risk of pregnancy practice contraception and 4% use the IUD. In Paraguay, 27% of women at risk use contraception, 6.7% using the IUD. In Peru, only 1% of the women at risk practice contraception, and 4% have an IUD.

In summary, of the South American countries, IUD use is widespread in Chile, Colombia, and Paraguay.

CONCLUDING REMARKS

France ranks highest in contraception rate (78.6%), second is the UK (74%), third is the USA (68%) and fourth is Spain (52%). The contraceptive pill is the preferred method everywhere except Latin countries, where the choice is still male withdrawal. The rate of IUD use in France is exceeded only by North European countries: Finland, Sweden, and Norway. Sterilization is rare in France and non-existent in Spain. In summary, in the industrialized countries the two modern methods of OC and IUD are the most common. The IUD is used by 20% of the fertile married women in Finland and Sweden. In Denmark, France, Japan, the USA, and the UK IUD usage is much less common. The pill may be dangerous to women aged over 40; the IUD is not so well tolerated by young women and the nulliparous.

Contraception in developing countries

Two-thirds of the world population live in developing countries. In 1990 one billion young people will have reached marriageable age. Attempts to delay the age of marriage have some effects on fecundity. 35% of couples practice some contraception worldwide; this percentage is reduced to only 20% in developing countries. In many countries, information is scarce and the demand for contraception is not met.

The measures taken during the past 5 years to decrease birth rate have had some effects, except in Africa, where family planning is nearly non-existent. Most countries, with the exception of those in Africa, try to reduce birth rate. In Asia and Latin America (e.g. India, Indonesia, Bagladesh, Thailand, and Brazil) international agencies provide funds for family planning programs, such as US AID (United States Agency for International Development), IFPF (International Family Planning Federation), WHO and UNICEF, the Population Council, and SIDA (a Swedish agency). Special efforts are made to dispense contraceptive products. In Sri Lanka and Jamaica pills are sold at retail prices.

IUD popularity

Among the millions of women practicing endouterine contraception world-wide, 13% live in industralized countries, 14% in developing countries and 73% in the People's Republic of China. Of the developing countries, Chile and Taiwan have the highest rates of IUD use, then Colombia, Egypt, South Korea, Mexico and Tunisia.

IUDs are rarely used in Africa: less than 1% of fertile married women use them in Kenya, Morocco, and Mauritius, and still less in Ethiopia and Zaire. In Hong Kong, Singapore, the Philippines, and Iran, 2–3% of such women use IUDs. 1% use them in Bangladesh, India, Pakistan, and Malaysia, and almost none in Afghanistan; in America the figure is 2–4%, as it is in Panama, Ecuador, the Dominican Republic, Nicaragua, and Costa Rica. 1–2% use IUDs in Salvador and Guatemala; the percentage is less in Haiti, Peru, Brazil, and Argentina. In some regions IUD use is made difficult by lack of information and qualified personnel. Kenya has increased the use of IUDs during the past 6 years. Since 1974, in 14 countries (Egypt, Mauritius, Tunisia, Afghanistan, Bangladesh, India, Iran, the Philippines, Taiwan, Thailand, Costa Rica, the Dominican Republic, Ecuador, and San Salvador), OC and sterilization have become popular. The OC rate is 10% in Venezuela, 8.4% in Brazil, 10% in Argentina, 7% in the Philippines, and 3% in India. The rate of injectable contraception in Colombia is 14%, in Costa Rica 24%, in Panama 18% and in the Dominican Republic 8%.

14
Use of IUDs in Latin America and Spain

B. VIEL

Among the many factors that influence the size of the birth rate in a given country, the percentage of fertile human couples practicing some form of contraception is one of the most important.

Table 14.1 shows the birth rate per thousand inhabitants in the years 1940 and 1975 in the Spanish-speaking countries. Spain, Argentina, and Uruguay, and to a lesser degree Cuba and Chile, were practicing contraceptive methods (condom, coitus interruptus, and illegal abortion) long before the present effective contraceptives were available. The rest of the Spanish-

Table 14.1 Birth rate per 1000 inhabitants in Spanish-speaking countries

	Birth rate		
Country	*1940*	*1975*	*% Reduction*
Spain	22.0	18.6	−16.5
Argentina	26.0	24.0	− 7.7
Uruguay	25.0	19.0	−25.6
Cuba	33.3	20.7	−36.4
Costa Rica	44.9	31.5	−33.2
Colombia	47.0	34.0	−26.1
Chile	33.4	25.0	−25.1
Panama	37.7	33.0	−12.5
Venezuela	43.9	36.0	−18.0
Dominican Republic	41.3	34.5	−16.5
Peru	47.1	41.6	−11.7
Ecuador	46.1	41.0	−11.1
Guatemala	45.2	43.2	− 9.2
El Salvador	49.1	43.7	− 7.3
Paraguay	43.0	39.8	− 7.4
Mexico	44.3	43.4	− 3.5
Bolivia	48.0	46.6	− 1.0
Nicaragua	42.2	46.0	+ 9.0
Honduras	37.1	48.0	+29.7

Source: Demographic Yearbooks

speaking countries in 1940 showed such high birth rates that the use of contraceptives was minimal and was restricted to the upper-class and higher middle-class groups.

There is no evidence that important migrations or major changes in the age distribution of the population, nor the age at which sexual life begins, have occurred during the last 35 years in the 19 Spanish-speaking countries considered. Illegal abortion may have increased during that period, but since it is illegal it is impossible to measure. With this sole exception, the significant decline in the birth rate in ten of the 19 countries compared in Table 14.1 should chiefly be attributed to greater availability and greater use of modern contraceptives, especially oral contraceptives (OCs) and IUDs.

It is not possible to ascertain with any reasonable degree of accuracy how much the use of IUDs has contributed to the decline in the birth rate. Only an indirect estimation can be obtained from those countries in which clinics supported by IPPF maintain records of the number of new acceptors. Table 14.2 shows the number and percentage of new acceptors of IUDs in the total number of new acceptors in the year 1977 in some of the Spanish-speaking countries.

Table 14.2 Proportion of IUD acceptors among new contraceptive acceptors in Spanish-speaking countries

Country	*Total no. of new acceptors*	*Total no. of IUD acceptors*	*Percentage*
Chile[a]	265 802	186 366	70.1
Colombia	59 478	30 871	51.9
Ecuador	7 014	4 566	65.1
El Salvador	47 514	8 252	17.4
Guatemala	11 547	1 776	19.8
Mexico	41 974	8 311	19.8
Costa Rica	22 641	435	1.6

[a] Chile reports the results obtained in a national programme. The rest reported results from private programs
Source: IPPF, Western Hemisphere Region, 1977

From Table 14.2 it is easy to see that in Latin America the use of IUDs varies considerably from one country to another. In Spain, according to a national survey of 1978 reported by Roncales (1979), only 1.0% of the couples practicing contraception were using an IUD.

All the follow-up surveys measuring active period of use by life table techniques show that the percentage still using a method of contraception at the end of 3 years is much greater among IUD users than among users of any other method. While in Chile carrying out a 3-year follow-up of 14 579 women inserted with Lippes D, I found the results shown in Table 14.3.

Since then a second and a third generation of IUD has been available. Thanks to these a considerable reduction in the expulsion rate as well as in removal for medical reasons has been obtained. Now, with an active IUD in multiparous women, continuation rates over 80% at the end of 3 years can

Table 14.3 Results of follow-up of 14 579 women fitted with Lippes D IUDs

Months after insertion	*Rate of:*		*Removal rate*		*Continuation rates*
	Pregnancy	*Expulsion*	*Medical reason*	*Personal reason*	
12	1.7	7.9	2.6	3.6	84.2
24	3.2	9.6	4.2	6.8	76.2
36	4.4	10.8	6.4	11.5	66.9

From Viel (1970).

be expected. The fact that active IUDs have to be periodically replaced should not be considered a disadvantage. On the contrary, the act of replacement could be an excellent opportunity for a clinical check-up and early diagnosis of gynecological diseases.

Follow-up studies of pill users in Latin America show a drop-out rate as high as 50% at the end of 1 year. Since hormonal oral contraception requires a great degree of discipline, it is possible that drop-outs could be less in groups with a higher educational background. No comparative studies of such a nature have yet been reported. Available evidence suggests that the IUD, although having a slightly higher associated incidence of pregnancies than the pill, should be considered the best reversible contraceptive available for people who live in the under-developed world, because of its high continuation rate.

The fact that in most Spanish-speaking countries the pill is more used than IUD can hardly be attributed to the preference of the users. There are no such differences between Chilean and Costa-Rican women. I am convinced that the preference lies with the medical profession. Medical doctors have not been properly trained (contraception is a subject very seldom discussed at the medical schools). Because they have not been trained they find it easier to prescribe than to insert. Since they do not recommend the IUD its availability is limited, and in countries where there are no Government-supported programs, the price of IUDs in the hands of the few who are able to insert them becomes exorbitant.

The medical schools bear enormous responsibility for the present reluctance to use IUDs more widely in under-developed Latin America. If medical students and auxiliary personnel were properly trained the use of IUDs would increase and the great opportunities for post-partum and post-abortion insertions would not be missed as they are today.

In countries where abortion is illegal a high proportion of maternal mortality arises from complications of self-induced or improperly performed abortion. There is evidence that women who have resorted to illegal abortion tend to repeat it if they become pregnant again (Requena, 1968). To protect such women from unwanted pregnancies will reduce maternal mortality and will also reduce the pressure on obstetric hospitals, where at present 30% of the beds are occupied by patients suffering from complications of illegally performed abortions. To insert an IUD immediately after curettage would protect these women and would not prolong the surgical intervention for more than 3 minutes. Goldsmith

(1972) has proved that such a procedure is safe and that the rate of expulsion is almost as low as that observed after menstrual insertion in normal women.

The insertion of Lippes D IUDs immediately after the expulsion of the placenta is a very good way to increase spacing. It has the inconvenience of a high rate of expulsion during the first month after insertion. In my own experience (Viel, 1970) based on 1228 post-partum insertions, 19% expulsion was confirmed at the end of the first month. After that the rate of expulsion was no greater than that observed with menstrual insertion. Re-insertion in those who suffered expulsion was successful and corrected the problem. The development of a Lippes D IUD secured with a catgut knot by Laufe (IFRP) has considerably reduced the early expulsion rate of post-partum insertions and made the procedure highly recommendable.

To increase the use of IUDs throughout the world, especially in the under-developed world where it shows a better continuation rate than other methods, two steps are essential. One is the proper training of medical students and midwives; the other, closely related to the former, is to increase availability. To increase availability, I recommend that the local manufacture of IUDs within user countries should be encouraged, especially in those that are far away from existing factories.

References

Goldsmith, A. (1972). Immediate post abortal intrauterine contraceptive device insertion. *Am. J. Obstet. Gynecol.,* **112**

Requena, M. (1968). The problem of induced abortion in Latin America. *Demography*, **5**

Roncales, J. M. (1979). Plantificación familiar en España. Presented at the *Medicated IUD Symposium, Spanish Session. Amsterdam, 1979*

Viel, B. (1970). Analysis of three years' experience with intrauterine devices among women in the Western area of the city of Santiago. *Am. J. Obstet. Gynecol.*, **106**

15
Use and regulation of non-physician health practitioners in family planning in the United States

S. SHARRETT

In 1970 the US Family Planning Act appropriated financial support to deliver family planning services to medically indigent women. However, it did not make available the medical personnel to carry out these services. In 1971, the Secretary of the United States Departments of Health, Education and Welfare (HEW) submitted to Congress a 5-year plan for family planning services and population research programs (Secretary of HEW, 1971). During those years an estimated 18 million women were in need of family planning services. Earlier shortages of physicians in the USA prompted the investigation of non-physician health professionals as a means of supplying family planning services (Surgeon General's Consultant Group, 1959). The American Medical Association supported this investigation by stating: 'The physician may properly delegate technical procedures to an allied health worker' (*American Medical News*, 1970). In 1971 Clyde Randall, president of the American College of Gynecologists and Obstetricians (ACOG) stated: 'The physician cannot personally provide all the needed health services. Physicians should begin to direct non-physicians to perform these routine tasks' (Randall, 1971). In 1973, Keith Russell, as president of ACOG, indicated that the College should adopt as one of its goals the proper development of the training and utilization of allied health professionals (Russell, 1973).

REGULATORY CHANGES

By 1975, 30 of the 50 states had amended their nursing practice Acts to facilitate an expanded nursing role (Bullough, 1975) and 37 states had enacted legislation authorizing the functions of physicians' assistants, who were originally medical corpsmen discharged from the armed services (Bullough, 1976; Dean, 1973). In addition, by 1976, 45 states and the District of Columbia had authorized nurse-midwives to handle normal deliveries (Forman and Cooper, 1976).

The changes in the expansion of licensure for nurse practitioners and nurse-midwives and in legislation licensing physicians' assistants were of critical importance to the organization and provision of family planning services. This created an enormous pool of family planning practitioners who could enhance the quantity and quality of family planning programs.

STUDIES OF CLINICAL TRAINING

In 1972, Ostergard and Broen, at Harbor General Hospital in California conducted a comparative study of IUD insertions by physicians and paramedical personnel (Ostergard and Broen, 1973). The trainees who had completed 14–24 weeks of formal training were composed of midwives, registered nurses, public health nurses, licensed vocational nurses, medical assistants, and individuals with no previous medical experience. Table 15.1 shows the results of the study: there were no significant differences between the physicians and non-physicians. For the non-physicians the life table event rates and complications were comparable with those achieved by the physicians. No perforations occurred in patients treated by either group and the incidence of subsequent pelvic inflammatory disease was similar for the two groups. Ostergard and Broen concluded that paramedical personnel with varying levels of previous medical experience can safely insert intrauterine devices.

Table 15.1 Insertion of Dalkon Shields by physicians and new health personnel (NHP): data computed by life table method for one year of use

Size of shield	*Category of personnel*	*No. of insertions*	*Women-months*	*Accidental pregnancy*	*Expulsion*	*Removal*		*Continuation rate*
						Medical	*Personal*	
Small	Physician	214	1416	2.4	5.7	17.4	2.7	71.8
	NHP	619	2898	1.4	3.9	9.8	3.5	81.4
	Overall	833	4314	2.1	4.2	13.3	3.3	77.0
Standard	Physician	301	2480	3.4	3.9	10.6	3.8	78.2
	NHP	1047	7741	0.9	2.7	8.8	2.2	85.3
	Overall	1348	10221	1.5	3.1	12.3	2.7	80.4

From Ostergard and Broen (1973).

Another study was designed to test competency of the non-physician providers and patient acceptance (Ostergard *et al.*, 1972). During a 44-week period in which 11373 patient visits were made, the registered nurse family planning specialist provided services to 88% of the patients without need for a physician's consultation. Family planning specialists without nursing degrees provided services to 80% of the patients without consultation. Of the patients referred to physicians, abnormalities were confirmed in 92–95% of the cases. Table 15.2 illustrates the degree of patient acceptance of non-physician providers in a study of 10582 IUD acceptors.

Table 15.2 Patient acceptance of the provision of family planning services by non-physician personnel. A survey of 10582 patients

Acceptance	*Percentage*
Prefer family planning specialist	43.8
No preference	55.6
Prefer physician	0.6

From Ostergard *et al.* (1972)

REPORTS ON CLINICAL PRACTICE

In 1973, an estimated 6% of approximately 46000 IUD insertions were carried out by non-physician practitioners in all ten regions of the USA (Kahn and Tyler, 1975). This indicates that an interpretation of medical-nursing practice laws permitted non-physicians to perform IUD insertions. Although no data are available on the types of non-physicians who performed these insertions, presumably the majority were nurses.

In 1977, R. Roemer indicated that in 1974, 108 of the 172 Planned Parenthood affiliates which provided medical services employed 207 nurse practitioners. Their clinical responsibilities were found to be related to medical policy rather than to legal barriers (Manisoff and Davis, 1975). Also surveyed were ten State Health Departments who replied that family planning nurse practitioners were employed at local health departments ranging in number from three to 30. They supplied a wide range of functions that depended on the judgments of the physician responsible for the clinic (R. Roemer, 1977). Both the Planned Parenthood and the State Health Department surveys indicated that nurse practitioners inserted and removed intrauterine devices (IUDs). Moreover, all indications were that the nurse practitioners performed these functions competently and to the satisfaction of both the physicians and patients.

GOVERNMENTAL PROJECTIONS

The Health Resources Administration of HEW has provided data for the numbers of nurse practitioners and physicians' assistants in 1975, 1980, and for 1990 (Health Resources Administration, 1978) (Table 15.3). For 1980, there was a projected number of 11430 nurse practitioners with an estimated 'high' number of 29890 in 1990, and 7410 physicians' assistants for 1980 with a projected 'high' of 27700 for 1990.

Although in the early 1970s there was a shortage of primary care physicians in the USA, it is predicted that the supply will exceed the demand by 1990. According to projections from the Bureau of Health Manpower, HEW, 1978, one out of every 400 persons in the USA will be a physician by 1990. The National Academy of Sciences, Institute of Medicine, stated in 1978: 'Because of the projected rise in physician supply an increase in the training rate of nurse practitioners and physicians' assistants now appears

Table 15.3 Present and projected supply of new health practitioners

			1990		
	1975	*1980*	*Basic*	*Low*	*High*
NP	5100	11430	23030	15840	29890
PA	2540	7410	18520	13200	27700
Total	7640	18840	41550	29040	57590

NP = Nurse practitioners
PA = Physicians' assistants
From Health Resources Administration, HEW (1978)

undesirable.' It seems clear that the future of the new health specialist is dependent upon the future supply of physicians.

DISCUSSION

Efforts to decrease support for new health professional training programs will probably affect nurse practitioners less than physicians' assistants. 88% of physicians' assistants training programs are federally funded as compared with 69% for certificate nurse programs and 39% for master's degree of nurse practitioner programs (Miike, 1979). Nursing administration has been phasing out the certificate programs in favor of master's level programs. Therefore, nurse practitioners may be more immune to future cuts in federal support.

Physicians' concern about increased liability with regard to nurse specialists may have been over-emphasized. The new statutes serve to protect both the nurse and the physician by providing a means for delegating certain functions of medical practice. Malpractice insurance provides coverage for the expanded nursing function. The absence of litigation affecting the family planning nurse practitioner is worthy of note (R. Roemer, 1977). In California, however, some of the nurse practitioners trained to insert IUDs were reluctant to do so as they felt that unsettled legal questions made them vulnerable to malpractice suits. Therefore, a more comprehensive legal reform is needed (Paxman *et al.*, 1976).

The wisdom of promoting the nurse practitioner as a doctor-substitute with the authority to diagnose and treat is questioned by some authorities. M. Roemer (1977) stated that such individuals may become substitutes for doctors only to provide care for the poor. None the less, advocates of the women's rights movement object to what they perceive as unnecessary control by predominantly male physicians over predominantly female non-physician specialists.

Non-physician family planning specialists play a minor role in providing family planning services in the USA. The expanded use of family planning practitioners depends on the willingness of physicians to delegate medical procedures to practitioners who are trained and competent. If the physician is unwilling to delegate some of his functions, he may be utilizing his skills less efficiently and limiting public access to family planning services.

CONCLUSION

It is interesting to note that 10 years ago there were major efforts to expand the role of non-physician health practitioners. Many cost-effective programs were instituted with favorable results. Yet, today, support for non-physician health practitioners appears to be diminishing. Apparently, many Americans are willing to pay more for training physicians, only to have them function at levels which utilize less of their medical expertise. Nurse practitioners have much to offer in the area of family planning; undoubtedly, they will not willingly remise their expanded professional roles.

References

American Medical News (1970). July 5, p. 6

Bullough, B. (1975). *The Third Phase in Nursing Licensure: The Current Nurse Practice Acts*, p. 153. (New York: Appleton-Century-Crofts)

Bullough, B. (1976). The law and the expanding nursing role. *Am. J. Public Health*, **66**, 249

Dean, W. J. (1973). State legislation for physicians' assistants: A review and analysis. *Health Services Rep.*, **88** 3

Forman, A. M. and Cooper, E. M. (1976). Legislation and nurse-midwifery practice in the USA. *J. Nurse-Midwifery*, **21**, 2

Health Resources Administration, US Departments of Health, Education and Welfare (1978). *Supply and Distribution of Physicians and Physician Extenders*, DHEW Publication No. (HRA) 78–11, Table 20, GMEMAC Staff Paper, prepared for the Graduate Medical Education National Advisory Committee. (Washington, D.C.: DHEW)

Kahn, H. S. and Tyler, C. W. Jr. (1975). IUD insertion practices in the United States and Puerto Rico, 1973. *Family Planning Perspectives*, **7**, 209

Manisoff, M. and Davis, L. W. (1975). Family planning nurse practitioners in the United States. *Family Planning Perspectives*, **7**, 154

Miike, L. (1979). The future of new health practitioners. *Family and Community Health*, **2**, 65

National Academy of Sciences, Institute of Medicine (1978). *A Manpower Policy for Primary Health Care*, p. 6. (Washington, D.C.: National Academy of Sciences)

Ostergard, D. R. and Broen, E. M. (1973). The insertion of intrauterine devices by physicians and paramedical personnel. *Obstet. Gynecol.*, **41**, 257

Ostergard, D. R., Broen, E. M. and Marshall, J. R. (1972). The family planning specialist as a provider of health care services. *Fertil. Steril.*, **23**, 505

Paxman, J. M., Lee, L. T. and Hopkins, S. B. (1976). *Expanded Roles for Non-Physicians in Fertility Regulation: Legal Perspectives*, Vol. 41, p. 47. Law and Population Monograph Series, Law and Population Programme. (Tufts University, Medford, MA: The Fletcher School of Law and Diplomacy)

Randall, C. L. (1971) *Inaugural address*. Presented at the *Nineteenth Annual Meeting, American College of Obstetricians and Gynecologists*, San Francisco,

Roemer, M. I. (1977). Primary care and physician extenders in affluent countries. *Int. J. Health Services*, **7**, 545

Roemer, R. (1977). The nurse practitioner in family planning services: Law and practice. *Family Planning Population Reporter*, **6**, 28

Russell, K. P. (1973). The ACOG, ten goals in 10 years. *Obstet. Gynecol.*, **42**, 637

Secretary of Health, Education and Welfare (1971). *Five Year Plan for Family Planning Services and Population Research Programs*. (Washington D.C.: U.S. Government Printing Office)

Surgeon General's Consultant Group on Medical Education (1959). *Physicians for a Growing America*, United States Public Health Survey, No. 709. (Washington D.C.: U.S. Government Printing Office) 1959

16
Family planning training centers for paramedical personnel in the Western hemisphere

R. WEINSTEIN

The International Planned Parenthood Federation (IPPF) is an international non-governmental organization made up of national family planning associations. The Western Hemisphere Regional Office, located in New York City, is responsible for providing technical and financial support for family planning programs throughout Latin America and the Caribbean. Among other types of training the Regional Office has co-ordinated over the years is medical and paramedical training. This includes programs for physicians in specialized surgical techniques, and for nurses and nurse-midwives in general contraceptive methodology. IPPF considers the latter type of training particularly important, because the organization has been promoting the utilization of non-physicians, especially nurse-midwives, in areas formerly ascribed to physicians.

Although most of the Family Planning Associations (FPAs) in our region are capable of providing basic training for standard family planning personnel, few are able to offer wide-scale training to sufficient numbers in the various disciplines used in family planning. To compensate for the deficiencies in local training, a number of countries are now offering training on an international or regional basis. I shall discuss types of program available throuhout the Western Hemisphere Region that are considered regional or international in scope.

First, for purposes of definition, 'international' programs are those which accept trainees from all parts of the world. For example, the Margaret Sanger Center in New York has trained nurses from Latin America, Africa, the Middle East, and the Caribbean. The scope of most training programs, however, is 'regional' in that trainees are accepted only from a particular region or group of countries, usually with the same or a common language. There are many centers which welcome nurses, nurse-midwives, auxiliaries, and other 'non-physicians', and which offer instruction in a variety of techniques.

All of the programs offer intensive, didactic instruction in contraceptive methodology and basic family planning skills. Most also include a practical component in which the trainee learns by working directly with clients or acceptors. The latter type provides fairly standard instruction in clinical skills, including conducting a physical examination (both pelvic and breast examination), taking Pap smears, inserting IUDs, fitting diaphragms, and distributing other contraceptive methods - pills, condoms, spermicides, foam and jellies. Trainees also learn to counsel and screen contraceptive acceptors. In addition, some programs provide instruction in urinalysis, blood pressure, and pregnancy testing.

Other skills are also taught, and these will vary depending on the needs of the particular population served by the training center. For example, part of the program at the University of the West Indies in Jamaica concerns the management of adolescent fertility. The Integral Family Planning Training Center in Chile emphasizes practical experience with rural and marginal populations. At Metropolitan Hospital in New York the emphasis is on family planning as part of a maternal and child health program. Almost all of the programs mentioned are designed to train nurses and auxiliaries to teach others; that is, to serve as 'trainers' themselves. Some also offer instruction in management techniques, and upon successful completion of the program the trainee should be able to serve in the administration of a family planning program.

These programs range from a 1- to 6-day basis and refresher course, as at the FPA in El Salvador, to intensive 16-week programs for nurse-practitioners at the Los Angeles County Harbor-UCLA Medical Center and the New Jersey College of Medicine and Dentistry. Another basic difference is that some programs award a certificate of successful completion, while others confer a title (e.g. Women's Health Care Nurse-Practitioner is used by Los Angeles County Harbor-UCLA Medical Center; Nurse-Practitioner or Nurse-Clinician is used by the New Jersey College of Medicine and Dentistry, Margaret Sanger and the University of California Extension at Santa Cruz).

Much has been written in the medical, population-related literature about the advantages of using paramedical personnel in family planning. To list but a few of these:

(1) They relieve the problems which result from the shortage of physicians, especially in rural or marginal areas.
(2) They relieve physicians from routine tasks, and once trained, paramedical personnel can carry out those tasks with a high degree of competency.
(3) They have a good rapport with clients, because they often come from the same community and social milieu, and speak the same language.
(4) Contraceptive technology has become sufficiently standardized and simplified so that paramedics can be trained to advise on and administer methods safely, inexpensively, and efficiently.

Unfortunately, despite these advantages and the availability of the types of training programs described above, nurses, nurse-midwives, and other non-physicians are often unable to use their skills when they return from their training because the supervisors or physicians to whom they report are unwilling to delegate responsibility to them. Often the physician feels threatened by the nurse's new-found skills and competence, and fears that she may assume some of his or her functions. In a study conducted in the English-speaking Caribbean of 27 nurses who had been trained abroad, it was found that despite intensive practice in insertion of IUDs, very few of the nurses were practicing this skill. Furthermore, very few had received salary increases or title changes upon returning to their countries.

One barrier to the effective utilization of these valuable personnel is that nurses and paramedics themselves feel inferior to doctors. They are in fact socialized into thinking that they are not as skilled or knowledgeable as the doctor. Such thinking is reinforced by social and class barriers. Often the nurse belongs to a different social milieu from the doctor or supervisor.

Nurses are also conditioned to serve as followers. They generally work under the supervision of doctors and tend *not* to be decision-makers. Thus, even if given the opportunity to make decisions about family planning, they may well defer to someone of higher authority rather than trust their own instincts. More than intensive training in family planning skills is required before such thinking can be reversed. There must be some basic change in long-held biases about medical skills and practice.

Several studies have been conducted in which nurses and other non-physicians, after appropriate training, have demonstrated a wide range of family planning skills as competently, and often more successfully, than comparable groups of physicians. When such studies have compared IUD insertions by nurses or paramedics with those done by doctors (e.g. Ostergard and Broen, 1973; Einhorn, 1978; Rosenfield, 1971; Delgado 1976), similar results have been achieved by both, with the paramedics occasionally producing a lower rate of expulsion than the doctor.

WHAT ROLE CAN THE NON-PHYSICIAN PLAY IN THE FUTURE?

Although there have been attempts to utilize the non-physician in other types of program (for example, to perform sterilizations or abortions) their acceptance by the medical profession, and by the institutions and communities in which they work, will depend on their demonstrated competence and the speed with which the law and both official and unofficial policy change to lend support to their efforts. Appropriate training is therefore essential, not only to give them the skills for performing procedures, but also for gaining stature in the wider community.

References

Delgado, G. I. (1976). Needs for training personnel in medical and clinical activities: a Chilean experience. In *Contraceptive Progress in Latin America and the Caribbean*. (New York: International Planned Parenthood Federation)

Einhorn, R. (1978). A Comparative Trial of Physicians and Nurses in the Delivery of Family Planning Services. *PhD. Thesis*, University of Colombia

Ostergard, D. R. and Broen, E. M. (1973). The insertion of intrauterine devices by physicians and paramedical personnel. *Obstet. Gynecol.*, **41**
Rosenfield, A. G. (1971). Family planning: an expanded role for paramedical personnel. *Am. J. Obstet. Gynecol.*

17
Research and new developments in intrauterine contraception

J. J. SCIARRA, A. SCOMMEGNA AND G. I. ZATUCHNI

The concept of intrauterine contraception has interested gynecologists since the early years of the twentieth century. It was not until the 1960s, however, that the intrauterine device (IUD) received wide acceptance by millions of women in almost every country of the world. In 1965, IUDs were being used by approximately six million women worldwide and 5 years later approximately 12 million women were using IUDs. By 1978, estimated users had increased to 50 million, the vast majority of them (73%) in the People's Republic of China. Of the remaining IUD users, 14% were in developing countries, and 13% were in developed countries (Ravenholt and Spiedel, unpublished observations). In the USA, IUD use has remained more or less stable in recent years at a level of around 6% or 7% of all contraceptors (Zatuchni and Sciarra, 1980).

HISTORICAL DEVELOPMENT OF IUDs

The first IUD, made of silk-worm gut in the form of a ring, was described in 1909 by Richard Richter, a European physician (Richter, 1909). Richter wrote that after many years of work, he had developed a simple, safe contraceptive that consisted of a silk-worm gut suture which could be inserted into the uterus. Irritation of the endometrium by the thread was so minimal that most women did not feel it, yet the device could prevent pregnancy. He reported that some women had used the device for almost 4 years. He found that insertion was easy; minor bleeding stopped after a few days, and removal was easily achieved by pulling the device out of the uterus with a forceps. After removal, fertility was restored. Richter's device was not well received by the scientific community, however.

In 1923, Karl Pust also described a ring made of silk-worm gut, but modified so as to include a tail fixed to a cervical button made of glass (Pust, 1923). This button was thought to serve as a mechanical barrier to spermatozoa and bacteria by closing the cervical os.

During the late 1920s, Ernst Gräfenberg developed an intrauterine ring composed entirely of silver coils. Because of his concern about possible pelvic infection, he opposed the use of any device having a thread or tail that might serve as a connecting bridge to the uterine cavity (Gräfenberg, 1930). In 1930, having fitted 600 women with the silver ring, he reported a 1.6% pregnancy rate and a 4% expulsion rate. Despite his favorable experience, and that of physicians in Japan, Denmark, Germany, and England using similar intrauterine rings, there was little enthusiasm for the intrauterine device during the next 25 years.

Several developments in the early 1960s led to the re-emergence of intrauterine contraception and the acceptance and use of IUDs by millions of women in almost every country of the world. Favorable reports on intrauterine rings made of silk-worm gut (Oppenheimer, 1959; Ishihama, 1959) prompted investigations into the use of modern plastics, metal, and other materials manufactured or molded into a variety of shapes and sizes. During that period, many world leaders developed an acute awareness of population growth rates, and researchers began thinking of appropriate contraceptive technology that could be used by the millions of women in need. It seemed that the establishment of national family planning programs, coupled with the promotion and use of intrauterine contraception, could provide the solution to the problem of increasing numbers of people.

IUD ACCEPTANCE AT PRESENT

Unfortunately, intrauterine contraception has not proved to be the solution to population problems that scientists and family planning experts had hoped. Except in a few countries - for example, Taiwan, South Korea, and Indonesia - the overall effect of IUD use on birth rates has not been substantial, owing to certain undesirable features of IUD use, as well as to cultural and sociological factors.

Major concerns with intrauterine contraception include danger of infection; undesirable side-effects (e.g. bleeding, pain, and expulsion); effectiveness; complications of use (e.g. anemia, perforation, neoplastic changes, spontaneous abortion, ectopic pregnancy, and congenital anomalies); restoration of fertility after removal; and non-medical factors, such as cost, ease of manufacture, and method acceptability. These concerns exist both for non-medicated and medicated intrauterine devices, although the possibility of neoplastic changes and congenital anomalies is more closely linked with devices utilizing copper or other metals and steroid hormones.

A number of confounding variables in published IUD studies make comparisons difficult and at times confusing. Since the clinical differences among most modern IUDs are small, such factors as age, parity, time of insertion, couple motivation, social and economic characteristics, clinic characteristics, insertion technique, and inserter experience may become very important in IUD comparisons with regard to pregnancy, bleeding, pain, expulsion, and other IUD-associated symptoms and signs.

Despite these problems, a contraceptive method requiring only one act of motivation from its user and then offering safe protection from pregnancy until the user wishes a return of fertility has great appeal; thus, investigators continue to seek out improved methods of intrauterine contraception.

PROMISING NEW DEVELOPMENTS IN INTRAUTERINE CONTRACEPTION

Various intrauterine delivery systems for fertility regulation are being considered; these include tubal closure substances, tubal motility activators, follicle maturation inhibitors, luteolytic substances, progesterone-receptor blocking agents, decidualization inhibitors, placental enzyme inhibitors, immunological agents, sperm enzyme inhibitors, and agents to alter cervical mucus.

Improvements in IUDs

Dissatisfaction with presently available metallic or plastic IUDs has prompted interest in the development of improved IUDs. Improvements should:

(1) Decrease the incidence and amount of abnormal uterine bleeding.
(2) Decrease the incidence of spontaneous expulsion.
(3) Decrease the incidence of pregnancy.
(4) Provide a new approach to fertility regulation.
(5) Provide certain therapeutic effects in addition to contraception.

In terms of meeting these objectives, one encouraging approach has been the addition of copper wire or sleeves to an inert plastic IUD. Problems with the wire copper-bearing IUD do exist, however. These include the possibly limited duration of effectiveness (perhaps only 3–5 years) and a potentially greater incidence of ectopic pregnancy; further, the safety risks among long-term users are unknown.

Incorporating steroids into the IUD has decreased the incidence and amount of IUD-associated bleeding and has lowered the expulsion rate; however, other problems have been noted with this approach, among them the relatively high pregnancy rates with progesterone-loaded IUDs, a worrisome increase in tubal ectopic pregnancies, and the possibility of abnormal embryonic development should a pregnancy occur in the presence of a steroid-loaded IUD.

Thus, the search continues for an intrauterine delivery system free of unwanted characteristics. Over the next decade, new IUDs may be marketed, but these are unlikely to be radically different from those that are presently being used; more likely, newer devices will include variations in design, such as shape, size, or geometry; modifications in copper configuration; or quantities and types of steroids loaded on the device.

Beginning research efforts are underway to develop IUDs for special uses during various times of the female reproductive life cycle. For example, the Lippes Loop has been modified with biodegradable wings on the upper arm to improve retention when inserted in a postpartum uterus immediately after delivery of the placenta or immediately after abortion. Copper devices have been inserted in women subsequent to unprotected midcycle intercourse to prevent implantation, should fertilization have occurred. Biodegradable devices are being considered for short-term use extending over a period of months.

Non-medicated IUDs

Empirical observations have indicated that an increased surface area of the IUD improves contraceptive performance, but large IUDs have often been associated with an increased incidence of removal for bleeding and pain (Figure 17.1). Currently used non-medicated IUDs represent a compromise in shape, size, and rigidity. An IUD such as the Lippes Loop is rigid enough to resist linear transformation so as to discourage expulsion, and yet will allow comfortable insertion through the undilated cervix.

Future developments in the physical properties of an IUD may improve retention. It has been suggested that retention rates are better with the more transversely flexible devices, possibly because transverse rigidity and longi-

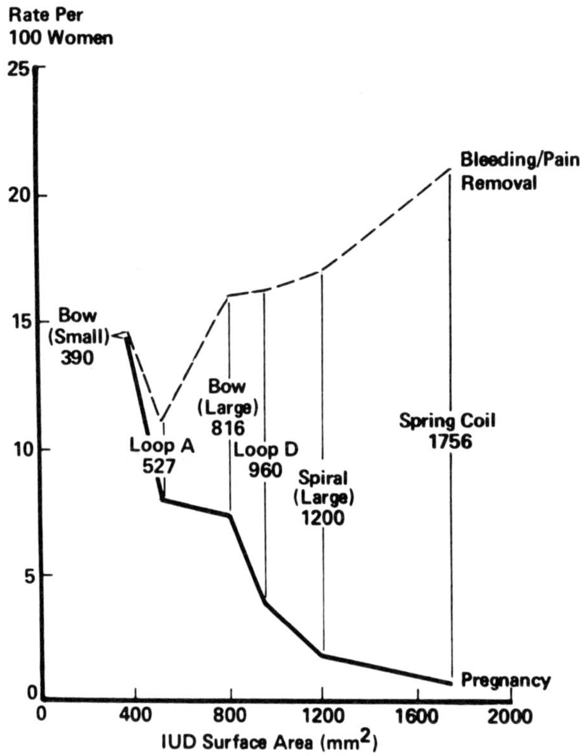

Figure 17.1 Rates of removal for bleeding and pain and pregnancy rates as a function of surface areas of IUDS (From *Intrauterine Devices.* Population Reports, Series B, No. 2, (1975), p. 43)

tudinal stiffness cause different uterine contractile patterns. The addition of small projections or anchoring fins similar to those used in the Dalkon Shield appears to improve retention of the T-shaped IUD.

Hasson (unpublished observations) has studied the relationships between uterine cavity and device lengths and has developed a prototype instrument capable of obtaining the exact measurements of the uterine cavity, including total length, length of the intracervical portion (external os to internal os), and the greatest and least widths. This type of uterine measurement holds promise for the selective fitting of IUDs, which would then assure accurate fundal placement, possibly increased effectiveness, and probably better retention.

Progesterone-loaded IUDs exhibit low rates of expulsion, as well as a low incidence of bleeding and pain. These properties are related to the smallness of the device, its shape and flexibility, and most importantly, to the effects of low doses of progesterone on uterine contractility. The addition of copper wire does not significantly improve expulsion characteristics; the lower rates of expulsion noticed with copper-bearing IUDs are related mostly to the size of the carrier. In a recent study, the addition of copper sleeves to a loop did not improve expulsion rates (Lippes and Jacobs, unpublished observations).

Improved IUD design may also lower the risk of pelvic inflammatory disease (PID). Organisms may gain access to the uterine cavity by way of the transcervical tail of the device. Most investigators feel, however, that IUDs with transcervical appendages do not pose a greater risk of infection than do untailed devices. Yet, in one study (Morris and Elstein, 1968) a tenfold decrease in the incidence of PID was seen in women wearing IUDs which were totally intrauterine, as compared with women wearing tailed devices. In another series, bacteria were often discovered at hysterectomy in the uterine cavity of women who had used a tailed IUD, whereas bacteria were not present in the uterine cavities of women who had not used an IUD or who had used an IUD without a tail (Sparks *et al.*, 1979).

The tail of the IUD has a dual function; it helps the woman to ascertain the presence of the IUD in the uterus, and it facilitates IUD removal. If the tail were demonstrated to be responsible for PID, however, it could be readily omitted or constructed of a biodegradable material. The development of a biodegradable tail or filament destined to dissolve and disappear 3 months after insertion could be an important addition to intrauterine contraception. The presence of the IUD in the uterus could be determined by other techniques. For example, the Antigon F has a small magnet that indicates the intrauterine presence of the IUD (Fuchs *et al.*, 1974). Similarly, new IUD retrieval devices must be developed.

Hysteroscopy has been shown to be an excellent method for removal of the IUD with missing filaments (Valle *et al.*, 1977); however, the technique requires sophisticated instrumentation and considerable operative skill.

Aside from improvements in physical characteristics and in the area of selective fitting, as long as the non-medicated IUD must depend on surface area for its contraceptive effect, further development of non-medicated IUDs with *significantly* improved overall performance is unlikely.

Present and future research with medicated IUDs

Adding medications to the IUD for slow release within the uterine cavity over a sustained period of time offers the possibility of truly improving IUD performance. Small devices with dimensions closely approximating that of the uterine cavity, although they produce fewer side-effects than the larger devices, are often associated with high pregnancy rates; addition of a metal or hormone has been shown to increase their overall effectiveness. This is a most promising area for research and should lead to the development and testing of second-generation IUDs.

Current studies indicate that the duration of effectiveness of the medicated IUD will undoubtedly be extended. Copper sheaths and sleeves instead of, or in addition to, copper wire have been added to various IUDs. This permits use of considerably more copper, which is released *in utero* for more than 10 years (Tatum, 1976). Similarly, a Progestasert device capable of releasing progesterone for more than 3 years is undergoing multicenter clinical trials (Pharriss and Rowe, 1979). Intrauterine delivery systems releasing a potent progestin such as levonorgestrel, at doses much lower than progesterone, promise to be effective for 5 years or more (Pharriss and Rowe, 1979; Nilsson, 1979).

Progesterone-loaded devices produce some vaginal spotting, as with the systemic administration of progestin-only contraceptives, although the total amount of blood loss for each menstrual cycle is markedly reduced. While this continued vaginal spotting is annoying for some women, it is completely unacceptable for others and often results in discontinuation of the method (Figure 17.2).

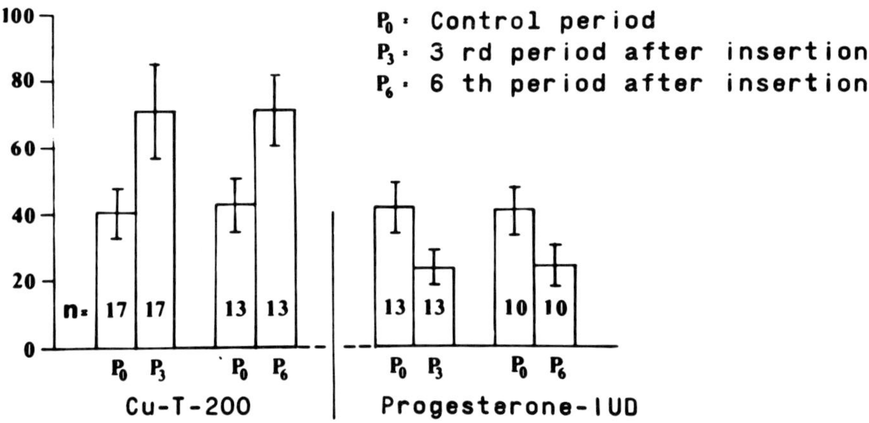

Figure 17.2 Comparison of menstrual blood loss with Progestasert System and Copper T (From Rybo, G., and Bergqvist, A. (1978). In Mishell, D. R. and Martinez-Manautou, J. (eds.) *Clinical Experience with the Progesterone Uterine Therapeutic System,* p. 106. (Amsterdam: Excerpta Medica)

An IUD with estrogen added is now being tested (Dmowski *et al.,* 1976) since even small doses of estrogen added to oral progestins will markedly decrease the occurrence of irregular vaginal bleeding. A somewhat weaker estrogen, estriol, has been chosen as the steroid to be released in the uterine cavity by the IUD. Estriol is produced in increasing amounts during pregnancy, and hopefully will not have deleterious effects on the fetus, in case of IUD failure. This is an important consideration, and before clinical use of a new medicated IUD, teratogenic screening must be performed on each drug to be released by an IUD. An estrogen-loaded IUD may also prove effective in preventing the reformation of uterine adhesions after the division of such adhesions by hysteroscopy in patients with Asherman's syndrome. A high estrogen dose delivered directly to the endometrium would encourage endometrial proliferation and accordingly discourage the reformation of adhesions.

Another approach presently undergoing investigation is the local release of a medication to treat IUD complications such as bleeding. The drug treats the side-effect, rather than increasing contraceptive effectiveness of the IUD. Overall effectiveness is thus enhanced because of fewer removals for bleeding. Although the cause of vaginal bleeding associated with IUD use is not clearly understood, one of the mechanisms used may be the increased vascularity with congestion, edema, and hemorrhage in areas of the endometrium not in contact with the IUD (Moyer and Mishell, 1971). These lesions may be responsible for the intrauterine activation of the plasminogen–plasmin system and its interference with the normal coagulation processes at the endometrial level. Women treated systemically with the antifibrinolytic substance tranexamic acid showed a marked decrease in uterine bleeding after IUD insertion (Westrom and Bengtsson, 1970).

IUDs releasing antibleeding agents or protease inhibitors are undergoing clinical trials (Tauber *et al.*, 1979). Preliminary evidence, however, indicates that interference with the fibrinolytic activity of the IUD may decrease its effectiveness. Some investigators have reported a reversal in the antifertility effect of the foreign body in rabbits locally treated with ϵ-aminocaproic acid (Srivastava *et al.*, 1979).

Newer medicated IUDs hold great promise for improving the overall performance of conventional devices.

New directions for IUD research

Future developments in medicated IUDs will be dictated by our increased understanding of reproductive physiology. As the processes of sperm migration, capacitation, and implantation are better understood, this increased knowledge will suggest ways to interfere with such essential reproductive processes. Prostaglandins play a multifactorial role in implantation. Recent evidence indicates that the following events essential for implantation are prostaglandin-related: fluid accumulation by the blastocyst, change in the permeability of maternal capillaries near the blastocyst, the decidual reaction, and the accumulation of prostacyclin in the myometrium at the site of implantation (Biggers *et al.*, 1981). Since prostaglandins play a role in several components of the implantation process, locally released prostaglandin antagonists or inhibitors of prostaglandin synthetase are likely to exert a very high contraceptive effect. Medicated IUDs releasing a prostaglandin antagonist or inhibitors of prostaglandin synthetase may be a particularly attractive form of contraception (Biggers *et al.,* 1978).

An exciting possibility is that a device of this type may be associated with a marked decrease in IUD side-effects. Because antiprostaglandins suppress uterine motility and decrease menstrual cramps, it is reasonable to expect an improvement in IUD retention rates with a decrease in IUD-related pelvic pain in such an IUD loaded with a pharmacologically active antiprostaglandin.

Continuous delivery of drugs by an IUD represents only the first step in the exploration of the many possible patterns of intrauterine drug delivery. Continuous delivery presupposes that the need for the drug is continuous throughout the reproductive cycle. We know that this is not the case. For an antifertility action directed, for instance, against the sperm, drug delivery would be necessary only when the spermatozoa traverse the uterine cavity. In a parallel fashion, an IUD carrying anti-zona pellucida antibody may provide an interesting new approach.

Special-use IUDs delivering tubal closure substances such as quinacrine are already in clinical trials (Goldsmith, unpublished observations). Such devices could serve the dual purpose of immediate intrauterine contraception and ultimate sterilization by tubal sclerosis.

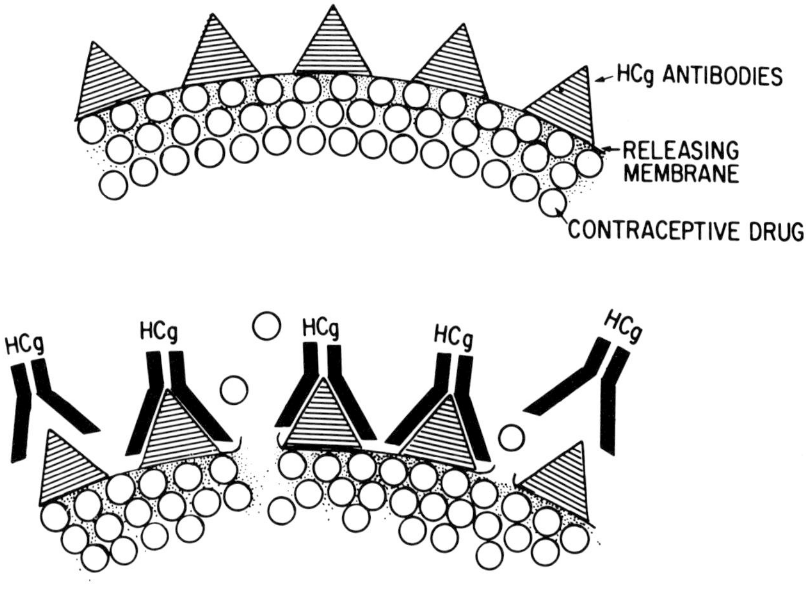

Figure 17.3 Hypothetical future IUD may use discontinued release. Release of contraceptive medication triggered by signal (HCG) generated by sperm or blastocyst (From Asch, R. H., Fernandez, E. O., Siler-Khodr, T. M. and Pauerstein, C. J. (1979). Presence of human chorionic gonadotropin-like substances in human sperm. *Am. J. Obstet. Gynecol.,* **135,** 1041

The ultimate intrauterine delivery system may be one whose critical component is a biological sensor capable of detecting and reacting to a biochemical or biological signal generated by the body itself. Drug delivery will then be self-regulated, dependent only on the body's need for the drug. Unfortunately, today very few sensing devices can detect and measure small amounts of biological substances present in a mixture as complex as the uterine or tubal fluid. Antibodies are both highly sensitive and highly specific chemical detectors. Thus, by incorporating appropriate antibodies into specifically-designed IUDs, the specificity and sensitivity necessary for detection in self-regulated drug delivery systems may be achieved.

In the hypothetical medical IUD of the future, human chorionic antibodies may be used in such a sensing device, so that contraceptive drug delivery will take place only when an egg has undergone fertilization, and not at other times (Figure 17.3). The future for development of pharmacologically active IUDs is very exciting, and such devices promise a whole new era of intrauterine therapeutics.

CONCLUDING REMARKS

Fertility regulation provided by a non-medicated IUD represents merely the initial step in the ultimate development of entirely new modalities of contraceptive therapy. Over the past half century, attitudes about the potential for intrauterine delivery systems of contraception have fluctuated from great optimism to overall rejection of the method. At present, physicians and researchers are gaining the perspective and experience to assess the value of this method of fertility regulation more accurately. Preliminary results of research and clinical experience now indicate the feasibility and usefulness of a wide variety of intrauterine delivery systems for enhanced fertility regulation.

References

Biggers, J. D., Leonov, B. V., Baskar, J. F. and Fried, J. (1978). Inhibition of hatching of mouse blastocysts in vitro by prostaglandin antagonists. *Biol. Reprod.*, **19**, 519

Biggers, J. D., Baskar, J. F. and Torchiana, D. F. (1981). Reduction of the fertility of mice by the intrauterine injection of prostaglandin antagonists. *J. Reprod. Fertil.* (In press)

Dmowski, W., Auletta, F. and Scommegna, A. (1976). Intrauterine release of estriol for contraception. Part I. In vivo results. In *Proceedings on Drug Delivery Systems*

Fuchs, F., Cederqvist, L. L. and Lauersen, N. H. (1974). The Antigon-F and the Ypsilon IUDs. In Wheeler, R. G., Duncan, G. W. and Speidel, J. J. (eds.) *Intrauterine Devices: Development, Evaluation, and Program Implementation,* p. 141. (New York: Academic Press)

Gräfenberg, E. (1930). The intrauterine method of contraception. In Sanger, M. and Stone, H. M. (eds.) *Practice of Contraception.* (Baltimore: Williams and Wilkins)

Ishihama, A. (1959). Clinical studies on intrauterine rings, especially the present state of contraception in Japan and the experiences in the use of intrauterine rings. *Yokohama Med. Bull.*, **10**, 89

Morris, N. G. and Elstein, M. (1968). Gonorrhoea and the IUCD. *Br. Med. J.*, **4**, 828

Moyer, D. L. and Mishell, D. R. (1971). Reactions of the human endometrium to the intrauterine foreign body. II. Long-term effects on the endometrial histology and cytology. *Am. J. Obstet. Gynecol.*, **3**, 66

Nilsson, C. G. (1979). Clinical trial with a progestin-releasing IUD. In *Proceedings of the International Symposium on Medicated IUDs and Polymeric Delivery Systems,* abstract No. 7.

Oppenheimer, W. (1959). Prevention of pregnancy by the Grafenberg ring method: A re-evaluation after 28 years' experience. *Am. J. Obstet. Gynecol.,* **78,** 446

Pharriss, B. B. and Rowe, P. (1979). Clinical experience with intrauterine contraceptive steroid delivery systems. In *Proceedings of the International Symposium on Medical IUDs and Polymeric Delivery Systems,* abstract No. 4.

Pust, K. (1923). Ein brauchbarer Prauenschutz. *Dtsch. Med. Wochenschr.,* **49,** 952

Richter, R. (1909). Ein mittel zur verhutung der konzeption. *Dtsch. Med. Wochenschr.,* **35,** 1525

Sparks, R. A., Purrier, B. G. A., Watt, P. J. and Elstein, M. (1979). IUD and pelvic inflammatory disease. In *Proceedings of the International Symposium on Medicated IUDs and Polymeric Delivery Systems,* abstract No. 31

Srivastava, K., Liedholm, P. and Astedt, B. (1979). Effect of epsilonaminocaproic acid (EACA) releasing IUD on implantation in rabbits. In *Proceedings on the International Symposium on Medicated IUDs and Polymeric Delivery Systems*, abstract No. 155

Tatum, J. H. (1976). Clinical experience with copper-bearing intrauterine devices and some thoughts on their mechanism(s) of action. In Moghissi, K. S. and Evans, T. N. (eds.) *Regulation of Human Fertility,* p. 194. (Detroit: Wayne State University Press)

Tauber, P. F., Hohlen, M., Zaneveld, L. J. D. and Ludwig, H. (1979). Antifibrinolytic agents for control of IUD-induced bleeding. In *Proceedings of the International Symposium on Medicated IUDs and Polymeric Delivery Systems,* abstract No. 52.

Valle, R. F., Sciarra, J. J. and Freedman, D. W. (1977). Hysteroscopic removal of intrauterine devices with missing filaments. *Obstet. Gynecol.,* **49,** 55

Westrom, L. and Bengtsson, L. P. (1970). Effect of tranexamic acid (AMCA) in menorrhagia with intrauterine contraceptive devices: A double blind study. *J. Reprod. Med.,* **5,** 154

Zatuchni, G. I. and Sciarra, J. J. (1980). Future developments in intrauterine devices. In Hafez, E. S. E. (ed.) *Medicated Intrauterine Devices.* (The Hague: Martinus Nijhoff)

18
Epilogue

W. A. A. van OS

The need for effective, safe, and easy-to-use contraceptives has not diminished with the advent of the contraceptive pill and the intrauterine device (IUD). Searching for total safety of conventional contraceptives continually stimulates new research. One approach to improving the effectiveness, safety, and acceptability is to develop methods of delivery that provide programmed medication. This is based on knowing that side-effects are generally dose dependent and that the degree of risk changes is in proportion to the dose. The preferred dose is one that evokes contraception with minimal risk.

The conventional delivery is by the oral administration and improved delivery is achieved by injectable depot formulations, non-biodegradable subdermal implants, capsules and rods, medicated intravaginal devices, medicated intracervical devices, biodegradable systems, and medicated IUDs.

A very promising feature of biodegradable systems is their possible utilization to achieve 'programmed' release. In the case of female fertility regulation, constant plasma concentrations of a steroid hormone do not allow maintenance of a regular menstrual pattern in all women. For this reason, pilot investigations are exploring the feasibility of constructing devices allowing pre-programmed release profiles, in which the active agent is made available only during specific periods. Medicated intrauterine systems represent a major advance toward achieving minimal intervention in fertility control.

The medicated IUD represents the first contraceptive system to focus on local, rather than systemic, delivery. The rationale for medical intrauterine delivery is based on the principle that drugs delivered directly to the uterine lumen in low doses will act directly on the uterine mucosa, inducing changes in the endometrium which prevent implantation. Supposedly, this can occur without influencing normal ovarian function and/or causing other systemic effects.

GEOMETRIC FACTORS

The geometric factors that reduce IUD performance are due to unfavorable geometric relationships between the IUD and the endometrial cavity (length, greatest transverse dimensions, anteroposterior dimension, surface area, and volume). Conditions at the time of menstruation produce a generally negative effect on IUD–uterine relationships. Unfavorable uterine characteristics include reduced luminal space, congenital fundal anomalies and uterine space-occupying lesions.

Because of their intrinsic limitation, non-medicated IUDs have failed to give continuation rates which differ significantly. An IUD with a greater surface area would always offer a low pregnancy rate and a higher removal rate because of metrorrhagia. The expulsion rate of IUDs has been inversely related to their stiffness. When stiffness is increased, expulsion rate decreases but metrorrhagia increases. Thus, the physical and biological properties required to obtain an optimal contraceptive result with low metrorrhagia and low expulsion rates are intrinsically opposed.

MODE OF ACTION OF MEDICATED IUDs

The extent and pattern of microvascular changes in the endometrium depend on the surface area of the IUD and the presence of copper or progesterone. In surface endometrial epithelium, a decrease in number of microvilli and a scarcity of cilia in ciliated cells occur. The physiological and clinical significance of changes in cell organelles is not known. The degree of ultrastructural change in the apical surface of cells is related to the age and parity of the patient, duration of period with the IUD *in situ*, and type of side-effect and complaint associated with the IUD. With 200 mm^2 of copper surface area, ultrastructural changes are noted in areas adjacent to the IUD. With a greater copper surface area, almost the entire endometrial cavity shows ultrastructural changes.

The following physiological mechanism has been implicated in the contraceptive action of IUDs:

(1) Disruption of the egg or sperm transport pattern.
(2) Changes in biophysical and biochemical characteristics of the endometrial fluid with subsequent inhibition of implantation of the blastocyst.
(3) Qualitative and quantitative alteration of oviductal and myometrial contractivity.

The mode of action of copper IUDs seems to include more than one of these effects. There is no evidence of any inhibition of ovarian functions and luteal activity through the hypothalamo–hypophyseal–ovarian axis; follicular maturation and the time of ovulation are normal in copper-IUD users. The contraceptive effect of IUDs is related to an endometrial foreign body reaction dependent on the surface of the device. Surface contact of the IUD with the endometrium is therefore one of the essential factors for the effectiveness. However, the contact surface of the newer copper IUDs

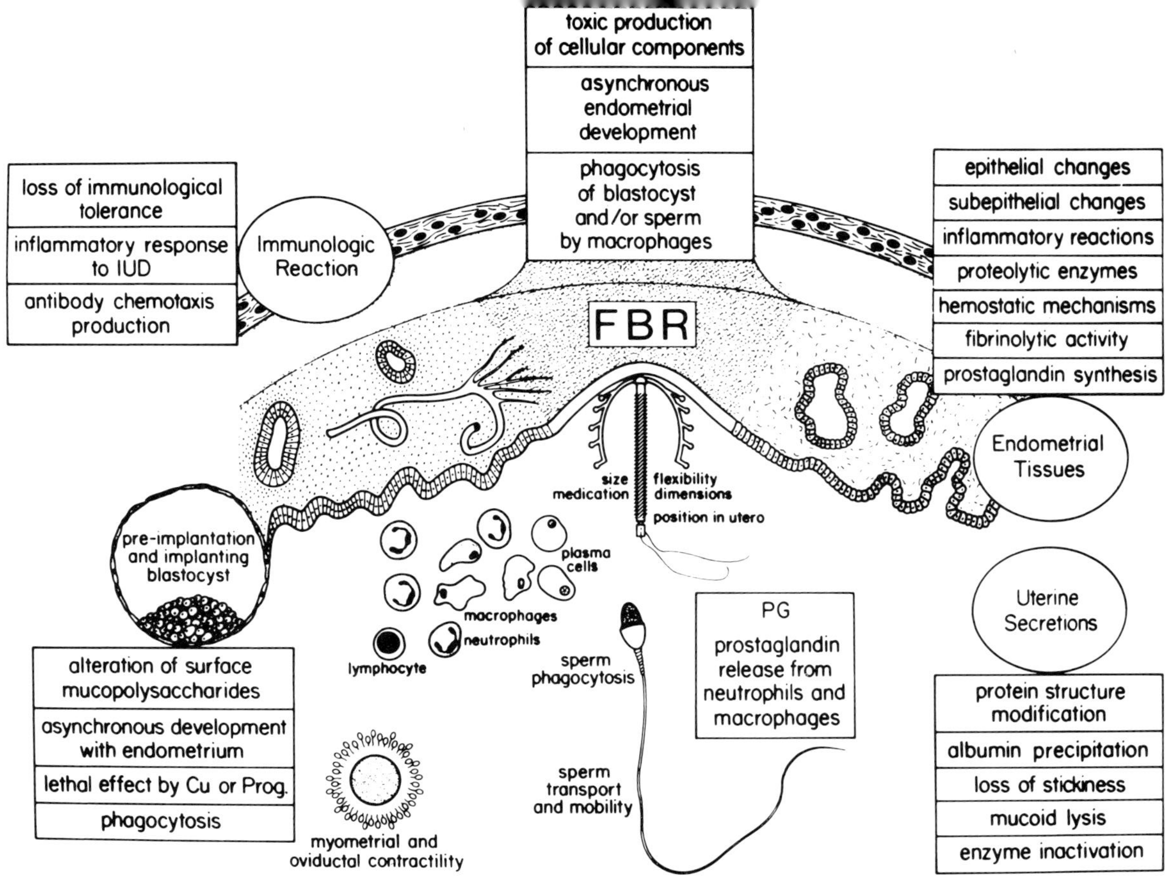

Figure 18.1 Suggested mode of action of inert and medicated IUDs. From El-Badrawi, H. H. and Hafez, E. S. E. (1980). Physiological mechanisms of IUDs, in Hafez, E. S. E. and van Os, W. A. A., *Medicated Intrauterine Devices*, p. 80. (The Hague: Martinus Nijhoff)

induces a stronger foreign body reaction, which is responsible for its contraceptive safety.

The additional substance added to the IUD – in this instance, the daily copper-ion release – is therefore required to spread over the surface of the endometrium distant from the device. It is therefore the copper ions that sufficiently modify the surface epithelium to prevent implantation. Clinical trials as well as scanning electronmicroscopy of the endometrium has proved that copper surface areas of 375 mm^2 result in a better contraceptive efficacy (Figure 18.1).

SPERM MIGRATION

Copper ions have a negative influence on sperm migration, but the migration is not completely prevented. The sperm migration disturbances can be considered as a partial effect in the multifactorial mode of action of IUDs.

The absolute production rates and the delicate balance between the different prostaglandins may be crucial elements in the development of side-effects and in the antifertility action of IUDs. There are remarkable changes in enzyme and metal contents of cervical mucus in patients with copper IUDs. Alkaline phosphatase used in energy production for the sperm may also be implicated in copper-device users.

The chemical state and the release rate of copper from the IUD are influenced by pH, oxygen tension, amount of blood loss, and protein components of the endometrial secretions. The contraceptive action of non-medicated and medicated IUDs depends on their ability to evoke inflammatory responses in the endometrium.

Non-medicated and copper IUDs cause an increased fibrinolytic activity in the endometrium. The secretory activity of the endometrial cells may be impaired. Myometrial contractivity is influenced by non-medicated and copper IUDs, whereas the addition of copper to *in vitro* systems alters the contractile activity of myometrial strips. Because *in vitro* copper interferes with the specific progesterone-binding capacity of human endometrial cytosol, one mode of action of copper IUDs may be that they interfere with progesterone at its target sites.

Copper IUDs do not inhibit sperm motility and metabolism except during the first months after IUD insertion when the copper concentrations are high in cervical mucus and endometrial secretions. The failure rate with copper IUDs decreases with increasing surface area of copper in the device, up to 375 mm^2.

MANAGEMENT OF IUDs

The correct IUD model should be carefully selected and adapted individually to all sizes of uteri. Devices too small or too large tend to be either expelled or increase the risk of unwanted pregnancies (Figure 18.2). More careful selection of the model should therefore be made before inserting an IUD.

Concern is evident when considering the risk of intrauterine translocation

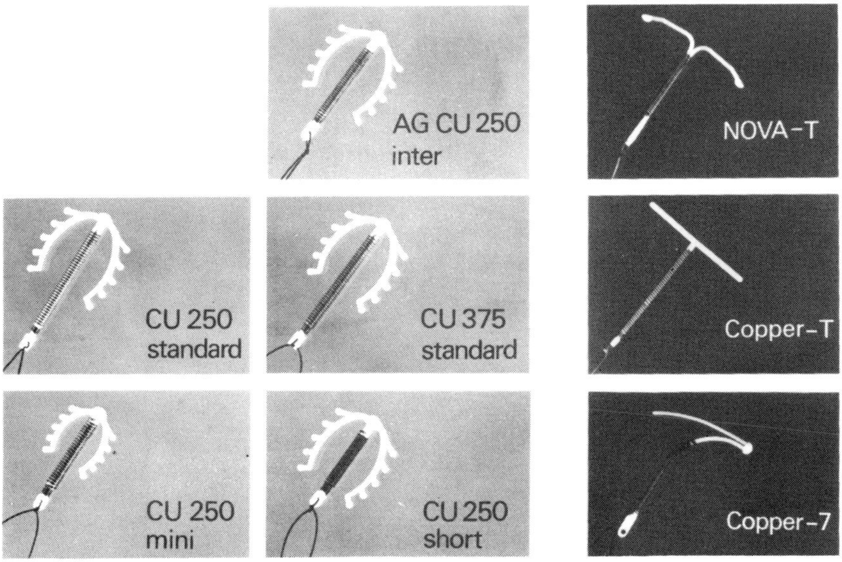

Figure 18.2 Different types of IUDs: Five Multiload models, Nova-T, Copper-T, and Copper-7

of the device, which could lead to erosion and subsequent uterine perforation. Comparatively, Multiload IUDs without lateral extension properties or a memory do not lead to the subsequent silent uterine perforation.

Efforts to improve the inserter, the insertion technique, and the device design have not solved the problem of postpartum expulsion. The use of biodegradables may create temporary architectural configurations which might improve IUD retention.

The following factors, in descending order, may be correlated with continued use of IUDs: parity, length of the cervix, length of the uterus, time from last menstrual period to insertion, length of menstrual cycle, previous contraceptive methods used, age, total number of abortions, additional children desired, and duration of menstrual flow. IUD insertion without a plunger is easier to perform, less dangerous for subsequent perforation, and preferable in developing countries.

PREGNANCY

Pregnancy can result from low positions of IUDs and inadequate contraceptive effects not related to position. Expulsion is caused by low IUD positions or excessive myometrial distension. Bleeding can be provoked by endometrial injury when the right size model for each individual uterus has not been carefully chosen.

Concerning factors in uterine perforation and displacement of the IUD, there are various physiological or pathological uterine conditions that weaken the uterine wall or hamper the access to the uterine cavity: the size, shape, design, and components of IUDs; and the plunger insertion technique of some devices are responsible intra-abdominally. Migration and subsequent visceral perforation depends upon the shape of the device and peritoneal irritation. Severe tissue reactions occur with copper IUDs.

IUD REMOVAL

The risk for removal because of infection of an IUD is dependent on age and not on parity. The degree of risk is two times higher than with other contraceptive methods and is seen relatively more often in younger patients. More research is needed to obtain further adequate scientific answers on this aspect.

ECTOPIC PREGNANCY

Any complaint associated with an IUD indicates an investigation for an ectopic pregnancy. The incidence of ectopic pregnancy among IUD users is related to age, gravidity, race, socio-economic status, and prior induced abortions. Most ectopic pregnancies are tubal, but the proportion of ovarian pregnancies is higher than in the general population. Women who become pregnant with any type of IUD *in situ* are at a slightly higher risk of ectopic pregnancy. In a pregnancy with an IUD *in situ*, the IUD should always be removed as soon as possible.

BLOOD LOSS

Increased blood loss in the IUD user is due to, amongst other factors, increased fibrinolytic activity of the endometrium as a result of the presence of a urokinase-like plasminogen activator. The fribrinolytic activity of the endometrium, not related to the stage of the menstrual cycle, is apparent in cases of dysfunctional bleeding. The inhibition of fibrinolytic activity explains the reduction of menstrual loss with the use of progesterone IUDs. Non-medicated and copper IUDs increase fibrinolytic activity at the superficial layer of the endometrium in contact with the device. The uterine fluid contains a proteolytic enzyme, probably an activator of plasminogen.

Progesterone-releasing IUDs give the endometrium a decidual-like appearance, and do not cause any increase in fibrinolytic activity in the endometrium. Intermenstrual bleeding during the first cycles, with frequent gradual decrease, is very small and does not cause a negative iron balance. This dysfunctional bleeding is probably due to mechanical damage to the endometrium. Device-induced dysfunctional bleeding can be treated by oral administration of synthetic antifibrinolytic agents – proteinase inhibitors (ϵ-aminocaproic acid [EACA], tranexamic acid [AMCA] and aprotonin [Trasylol]). The disadvantage of oral application of these inhibitors is the occurrence of unwarranted side-effects due to the large quantities that have to be given.

Progesterone-releasing IUDs improve contraceptive efficiency and alter menstrual bleeding patterns. The progesterone-releasing IUD causes various histological and cytological changes: chronic non-specific inflammation and irregular arrested shedding of endometrium; decrease in number of endometrial granulocytes; suppression of nucleolar channel systems and endometrial glycogen; decrease in number of ciliated cells in the endometrium; and increased lysosomal aggregates in the oviductal epithelium typical of the first trimester of pregnancy. Physiological responses with this device include decreased prostaglandin concentration in endometrium and menstrual blood, reduced myometrial activity, reduced menstrual blood loss, and reduced dysmenorrhea.

The effectiveness of intrauterine prostaglandins is related to their ability to induce decidual and suppressive changes in the endometrium. Endometrial changes may play a significant role in the mechanism of contraceptive action of intrauterine prostaglandins. Pregnancy rates with progesterone-releasing IUDs are less than two per 100 women per year for parous women and slightly more for nulliparous. The ectopic pregnancy rate is about 0.4 per 100 woman-years with regional variations as a result of variations in user characteristics and tubal damage due to previous pelvic inflammatory disease (PID). The rate of spontaneous abortions with the IUD *in utero* is 50%.

The levonorgestrel-releasing IUD, with a developer's expected lifetime of 5 years, causes a significant decrease in menstrual blood loss from 21 ml during treatment to 52 ml before treatment. The decrease in blood loss is associated with a significant increase in peripheral blood hemoglobin concentrations.

CLINICAL EVALUATION

Clinical evaluation of various medicated IUDs was noted with special emphasis to the efficacy, degree of side-effects, expulsion rates, and conformation rates. Some authors claim that IUDs last 3 years while others claim 5. Hopefully, multicentered randomized studies could be conducted to ensure the accuracy of such claims, since this will be of great advantage to developing countries, and more effort will be concentrated on the development of newer IUDs with simplified insertion techniques for the rural areas in developing countries. Measures of IUD performance - pregnancy, expulsion, removals for pain, bleeding, or other medical reasons - remain within the standard criteria for IUD evaluation. In addition, problems that are more rare - yet generally more serious than pain, bleeding, and expulsion - have now emerged so that long-term and widespread use has made it possible to detect rare events.

A copper wire of 0.225 mm diameter with a surface area of 200 mm^2 (Cu-T, Cu-7, and Nova-T models) provides an antifertility effect for some 2 years. A copper wire of 0.3 mm diameter with a surface area of 250 mm^2 (ML Cu-250 IUD) provides a better and longer effect for some 3 years. A copper wire of 0.4 mm diameter with a copper surface area of 375 mm^2 (ML Cu-375 IUD) shows a higher antifertility effect for the first 2 years of use. No evidence is yet available over a longer period. No fragmentation has appeared with 0.4 mm diameter copper wire.

The Nova-T furnished with silver-cored copper wire with a 200 mm^2

copper surface area is claimed to have an effective lifetime of 5 years. Unfortunately, conferring evidence for the 5-years lifetime is still lacking.

NEW CHANGES IN TECHNOLOGY

Porous polymers, avoiding a difficult membrane-controlled system, can hopefully achieve a simpler release of steroids or other drugs. The belief that estriol may have a contraceptive effect within the uterus by binding to estrogen receptors and hopefully not altering the normal uterine cycle is being extensively tested.

FUTURE METHODS

One way of considering non-surgical female sterilization is to develop the intrauterine delivery of a sclerosing agent at the uterotubal opening via the vaginal cervix and uterus. By irritating the tissue of the fallopian tube, the substance causes the lumen of the tube to close without scarring. Effectiveness should be as high as that experienced with current methods of surgical sterilization.

A post-placental medicated IUD has to be inserted immediately after delivery of the placenta. Conventional IUDs inserted during the postpartum period are likely to be expelled about three times more often than when they are inserted during the menstrual cycle. Ideally, such a device would be effective over a woman's entire reproductive lifespan, and would maintain effectiveness without being replaced for several years. Insertion by a specially trained non-physician birth attendant should be feasible.

Devices with biodegradable retentive components designed to reduce expulsion after immediate post-placental and post-abortion insertion are being developed and clinically tested. No firm evidence of effectiveness has yet been reported.

LEGAL AND ETHICAL CONSIDERATIONS

Government regulation of IUDs affects the worldwide availability of all contraceptives. Different countries have different risk–benefit ratios and demographic considerations. Developing and testing medicated IUDs with active ingredients such as copper, zinc, or steroids will raise more research issues and better mathematical models for clinical evaluations. Finally, making the results of extensive IUD research programs available to health professions, clinical centers, and national family planning programs will require a high degree of co-operation nationally and internationally.

Research networks will need to share protocols and experience; data will have to be fully available and openly discussed; manufacture of devices will have to be arranged at convenient locations providing good quality control and reasonable prices; and finally, distribution programs will have to provide adequate supplies and accurate clinical guidance on a large scale.

The greatest challenges in medicated IUDs development today may not only be technical improvement of devices and clinical procedures but also efficient dissemination of improved devices and equipment to programs that need them. Developing long-acting contraceptive systems requires the application of more sophisticated technology and wider diversity of technological expertise.

The new systems being developed require input from biomaterial specialists, life scientists, and clinicians. The multidisciplinary approach to research requires centralization of advanced expertise and a broad funding base in order to be totally effective. The current philosophy of government funding is, however, leaning in the opposite direction.

Appendix
IUD technology*

PATIENT MOTIVATION

The patient should indicate her preference for this method and should be informed of the effectiveness rates, as well as the potential side-effects associated with it. This is particularly important because the patient may experience minor side-effects in the first few months. Such side-effects may lead to early discontinuation, particularly in patients who have not received adequate instruction.

CONTRAINDICATIONS

The following should be given consideration as possible contraindications to the insertion of IUD:

(1) Major.
   (a) Pelvic infections (acute, subacute, or recurring).
   (b) Known or suspected cervical or uterine malignancy, including unresolved, abnormal Papanicolaou smears.
   (c) Pregnancy.
(2) Relative.
   (a) Uterine abnormalities such as congenital anomalies and myomas distorting the uterine cavity.
   (b) Hypermenorrhea.
   (c) Dysmenorrhea.

SELECTION OF DEVICE AND SPECIAL INDICATIONS

The uterus should sound to a depth of 6–8 cm. The patient whose uterus

* ACOG Technical Bulletin No. 40, June, 1976 (replaces No. 10, September, 1974). This bulletin does not represent official policy or recommendation of the American College of Obstetricians and Gynecologists, but rather describes methods and techniques of practice that are currently acceptable and used by recognized authorities.

measures less than this may require a smaller form of the IUD and the patient with a greater uterine measurement may require a larger device.

With the use of all medicated inrauterine devices, it is advisable to check the patient's known sensitivities. While the inert intrauterine device has no time limit, the medicated forms (including copper) carry appropriate expiration dates. This information should be clearly communicated to the patient.

Some early reports have indicated that the copper-bearing devices are effective in preventing implantation when inserted postcoitally. As is true for the use of estrogen in this circumstance, the sooner after exposure the IUD can be inserted the more effective the method seems to be.

In the case of Asherman's syndrome, once the synechiae have been broken up, the insertion of an IUD will often prevent their reforming.

SPECIAL CONSIDERATIONS

Patients with a history of valvular heart disease and patients with a susceptibility to infection (chronic consumption of corticosteroids, leukopenia, or leukemia, etc.) should receive appropriate antibiotics for a month following insertion of an IUD.

The use of an IUD in patients who are receiving anticoagulants or who have a coagulopathy may be contraindicated.

Postpartum insertions carry a higher risk of uterine perforation if carried out prior to the eighth week postpartum. For any individual patient this increased risk must be weighed against the risk of pregnancy, and the patient's co-operation in returning for subsequent appointments - as well as her willingness to use an interim form of contraception - must be evaluated. Insertions following a first-trimester abortion do not carry this increased risk.

PATIENT COUNSELING

To insure patient participation in the decision-making process as to her most appropriate contraceptive method, it is important to provide her with information covering the relative effectiveness of various methods, as well as their benefits and risks. Following appropriate consultation, examination, laboratory testing, and selection of the method, the patient should be informed about potential minor and major side-effects. She should be advised of symptoms, the occurrence of which may necessitate a problem visit or discontinuation of the method. Availability of medical care in the event of an emergency related to use of the contraceptive method needs to be clarified for the patient. Documenting the foregoing steps in the patient's record is recommended.

The overall failure rate (pregnancy) of approximately 3% or less (ranging from 1 to 5% depending on age and parity, as well as other factors) should be explained to the patient. Patients desiring a higher rate of effectiveness should be counseled to use additional methods at the time of presumed ovulation, particularly during the first 3 months. Approximately 25% of patients require removal or will spontaneously expel an IUD during the first year of use.

MINOR IUD SIDE-EFFECTS

In certain patients, paracervical block may be utilized to minimize insertional pain. Syncope may occur in patients with a previous disposition to this condition. Atropine may be given intravenously prior to insertion to decrease the incidence of bradycardia and vasovagal reaction. Other minor side-effects may be uterine cramps, intermenstrual bleeding, increased menstrual flow, and increased vaginal discharge.

TECHNIQUE OF IUD INSERTION

The technique of insertion varies with the type of device. In general the following steps are suggested:

(1) Bimanual examination should be done to ascertain the size, shape, and position of the uterus.
(2) If indicated, a gonorrhea culture should be taken from the endocervix.
(3) A Papanicolaou smear should be taken if not recently obtained.
(4) The ectocervix should be cleaned with an antiseptic solution.
(5) A tenaculum should be applied to the cervix with downward traction for correction of the angulation of the uterus and stabilization of the cervix.
(6) The cervical canal should be sounded prior to insertion for depth and direction of the uterine canal. In occasional cases, cervical stenosis may preclude the use of intrauterine contraception. Undue force should not be employed in an attempt to overcome this resistance. The instruments entering the cervical canal, as well as the IUD, must be sterile.
(7) IUDs should preferably be inserted during menstruation to reduce the chance of insertion into a pregnant uterus, as well as to facilitate the insertion. This approach may not be practical in all clinical situations.
(8) The risk of uterine perforation may be reduced by employing the withdrawal technique of insertion for those devices with movable cervical stops on the inserter. After sounding the uterus, the stop should be set so that the tip of the inserter is approximately 0.5 cm from the top of the endometrial cavity. The inserter is advanced until the stop is at the cervical os, the plunger placed against the bottom end of the device, and the sleeve is withdrawn over the plunger, depositing the device high in the uterine cavity.
(9) At the time of insertion, the patient should be taught to check for the string of the IUD.

CONTINUING CARE OF WOMEN USING IUDs

Since the pregnancy rate with the use of IUDs is slightly higher than with oral contraceptives, particularly during the first few months of use, patients unwilling to use abortion as a back-up procedure should be advised to use an adjunctive contraceptive method around the time of presumed ovulation.

Women should be re-examined within 3 months after insertion, preferably shortly after the first post-insertion menstrual period. Thereafter, annual examinations with appropriate medical and laboratory evaluations should be carried out.

If the string is visible and the IUD appears to be properly placed, it should be left undisturbed.

COMPLICATIONS

Acute pelvic inflammatory disease may develop. Some mild infections can be treated with suitable antibiotics with the IUD in place. If serious infection develops, culture and sensitivity should be obtained from the endocervix, including anaerobic culture, the device removed, and antibiotic treatment against anaerobes instituted.

The early symptoms of progressive endometrial infection occurring with an IUD are foul-smelling leukorrhea, premenstrual bloating, dyspareunia, intermenstrual bleeding, and hypermenorrhea. This can be relatively silent, of insidious onset, and is often first identified by the finding of a tender tubo-ovarian mass. Women developing these infections should have aerobic and anaerobic bacteriological studies of the cervical canal and uterus and indicated antibiotic therapy. Removal of the IUD is necessary. Early recognition and treatment of this complication may avert serious sequelae.

In addition to the conditions mentioned above, IUDs may also need to be removed for hypermenorrhea, abnormal bleeding, and intractable pain often aggravated by intercourse.

THE 'LOST' IUD

If a string of the IUD cannot be seen and the patient is not aware of the IUD having been expelled, three potential situations must be considered and explored:

(1) Pregnancy. This possibility must be evaluated in the usual ways (history, pelvic examination, and appropriate laboratory tests).

(2) Unnoticed expulsion. If there are no signs of pregnancy, the presence or absence of the IUD and its position must be determined using one or more of the following methods: probing the uterus for retracted string and/or the presence of the IUD, ultrasonography, posterior–anterior and lateral X-rays of the pelvis with the position of the uterine cavity indicated by one of the following techniques:
   (a) Metal uterine sound.
   (b) Radiopaque dye via catheter.
   (c) Insertion of another IUD of a different type.
   (d) Hysterogram.

(3) Perforation. Perforation is a known risk with IUD insertion. The perforation rate varies with the experience of the individual performing the insertion, ranging from 0.5 per 1000 insertions to 10 per 1000 insertions. Most reports indicate that the range of perforation is around 0.5–3 per 1000 insertions. In some instances

when perforation occurs at the time of insertion, it is immediately recognized. However, it may be partially initiated at the time of insertion, remain partial, proceed to a full perforation or become embedded in the uterine wall. Perforation of the cervix or lower segment of the uterus with the vertical arm of certain devices can occur spontaneously in a small percentage of cases. If the IUD is found to be outside the uterine cavity and free in the abdominal cavity, it should be removed by laparoscopy, culdoscopy, or laparotomy. If it is a copper-bearing device, this removal should be effected promptly because of the predisposition to the formation of dense adhesions.

IUD REMOVAL

A desired pregnancy or patient request are elective reasons for removal of an IUD. Indicated reasons for removal would include pelvic pain and/or cramping, abnormal bleeding, pregnancy (string visible), uncontrolled pelvic infection, and replacement of medicated device.

Simple removal of an IUD is usually accomplished at pelvic examination by traction on the string of the IUD with forceps. When difficulty is encountered with IUD removal, removal may be facilitated by any one or a combination of the following adjunctive measures: paracervical block, use of tenaculum on cervix to straighten cervico-uterine axis, use of polyp forceps, alligator clamp, or other instruments.

If the IUD is embedded in the myometrium, localization of the device (as above) is helpful. The degree of penetration and/or perforation will dictate whether the device is best removed by dilatation and curettage, hysteroscopy, or laparotomy.

MANAGEMENT OF THE IUD IN PREGNANCY

A complete evaluation is important in assessing any potential pregnancy with the IUD in place. Particular consideration should be given to the possibility of an ectopic pregnancy, as this occurs with relatively greater frequency in the presence of an IUD. Removal of the IUD when pregnancy is detected results in a reduction of spontaneous abortion from an expected rate of approximately 50% to about 25%. Removal also minimizes the risk of septic abortion, known to be a hazard when the IUD remains in place.

Intrauterine pregnancy with string visible

The IUD should be removed immediately if this can be done with ease and the patient referred for prenatal care or termination.

Intrauterine pregnancy with string not visible

It is important to determine whether the pregnancy occurred as a result of spontaneous, unnoticed expulsion or whether the IUD is still present, as well as the type of device. If the gestation is 10–12 weeks or more, the string of the IUD may have been drawn up inside the enlarging uterus. Ultrasonography for IUD identification is preferred, particularly when the patient may elect to carry the pregnancy. X-ray diagnosis may be necessary. If the IUD is present, an informed decision should be made by the patient with awareness of risks of all options whether to continue the pregnancy or elect termination. Prior to her decision, it is important that she be made aware of the increased hazard of septic abortion, including death (particularly if the device has a multifilament tail), if the pregnancy continues with the device in place. If the patient elects to continue the pregnancy, she must be closely observed. She should be advised to report all abnormal symptoms, such as flu-like syndrome, fever, abdominal cramping and pain, or bleeding, as symptoms may be insidious. Death has been known to occur within 72 hours of onset of symptoms. If symptoms suggestive of onset of mid-trimester septic abortion occur, aggressive treatment must be instituted. Steps must be taken immediately to evacuate the uterine contents. Concomitant antibiotic therapy, effective against anaerobes, must also be initiated. In rare instances, hysterectomy may be necessary.

Bibliography

Burnhill, S. (1973). Syndrome of progressive endometritis associated with intrauterine contraceptive device. *Adv. Planned Parenthood,* **8,** 144

Christian, C. D. (1974). Maternal deaths associated with an IUD. *Am. J. Obstet. Gynecol.,* **119,** 441

Mishell, D. R. Jr. and Moyer, D. L. (1969). Association of pelvic inflammatory disease with the intrauterine device. *Clin. Obstet. Gynecol.,* **12,** 179

Scott, R. B. (1968). A survey of deaths and critical illnesses in association with the use of intrauterine devices. *Obstet. Gynecol.,* **31,** 322

Tatum, H. J. (1972). Intrauterine contraception. *Am. J. Obstet. Gynecol.,* **112,** 1000

Tietze, C. and Lewis, S. (1970). Evaluation of intrauterine devices. Ninth progress report of the cooperative statistical program. *Stud. in Family Planning,* **55,** 1

Index

Progress in Contraceptive Delivery Systems

SERIES EDITOR E. S. E. HAFEZ

Other volumes in this series are detailed below:

Volume I **Biodegradables and Delivery Systems for Contraception**

Editors: E. S. E. Hafez and W. A. A. van Os

I. BIODEGRADABLES

1 Biodegradable delivery systems
W. E. Skiens, F. G. Burton and G. W. Duncan

2 The design of controlled drug delivery systems based on biodegradable polymers
C. G. Pitt and A. Schindler

3 Biodegradable microcapsules and microparticles for contraception
D. L. Gardner and D. J. Fink

4 Systemic and local delivery of contraceptive steroids using biodegradable micropasules
L. R. Beck, D. R. Cowsar and D. H. Lewis

5 Biodegradable cylindrical implants for fertility regulation
J. D. Gresser, D. L. Wise, L. R. Beck and J. F. Howes

6 Improving IUD performance with biodegradable materials
L. E. Laufe and P. G. Friel

7 Device design and system application
G. W. Duncan, F. G. Burton and W. E. Skiens

II. CONTRACEPTIVE DELIVERY SYSTEMS

8 Intratubal devices
J. Brundin

9 Medicated intracervical devices
F. G. Burton, W. E. Skiens, G. W. Duncan and M. R. Sikov

10 Contraceptive vaginal rings: mechanism of action and historical development
S. Roy and D. R. Mischell

III. EXPERIMENTAL APPROACHES

11 Development of bioerodable contraceptive insert
B. Pharriss and E. Schmitt

12 Agglutination, immobilization and phagocytosis of spermatozoa, and contraception development
E. S. E. Hafez

13 Epilogue
E. S. E. Hafez

ISBN 0-85200-345-5

Volume II **IUDs and Family Planning**

Editors: E. S. E. Hafez and W. A. A. van Os

I. POPULATION DYNAMICS

1 Introduction to family planning
Mrs E. Veder Smit

2 Human fertility and population dyamics
E. S. E. Hafez

3 Fertility regulation and family planning
E. S. E. Hafez

4 World experience with use of IUDs
J. J. Speidel and R. T. Ravenholt

5 The IUD: its role in the population programs of the developing world
A. Goldsmith, A. Beth Young and Christine E. Colven

II. FAMILY PLANNING IN EUROPE AND THE AMERICAS

6 IUDs and family planning in the Netherlands
E. Ketting

ISBN 0-85200-346-3

Volume III IUD Pathology and Management

Editors: E. S. E. Hafez and W. A. A. van Os

ISBN 0-85200-347-1